A Cup of Comfort® for Nurses

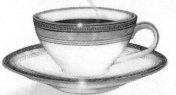

Stories of Caring and Compassion

EDITED BY
COLLEEN SELL

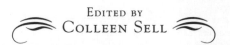

ADAMS MEDIA
Avon, Massachusetts

For Judy, nurse and friend extraordinaire

A Cup of Comfort. is a registered trademark of F+W Publications, Inc.

Published by
Adams Media, an F+W Publications Company
57 Littlefield Street, Avon, MA 02322. U.S.A.

www.adamsmedia.com and *www.cupofcomfort.com*

ISBN: 1-59337-542-5

Printed in Canada.

J I H G F E D C B A

Library of Congress Cataloging-in-Publication Data
A cup of comfort for nurses : stories of caring and
compassion / edited by Colleen Sell.
p. cm. -- (A cup of comfort series book)
ISBN 1-59337-542-5
1. Nursing--Anecdotes. 2. Nurses--Anecdotes. I. Sell, Colleen. II. Series.

RT82.C86 2006
610.73--dc22

2005026432

This publication is designed to provide accurate and authoritative information
with regard to the subject matter covered. It is sold with the understanding that
the publisher is not engaged in rendering legal, accounting, or other professional
advice. If legal advice or other expert assistance is required, the services of a
competent professional person should be sought.

—From a *Declaration of Principles* jointly adopted by a Committee of the
American Bar Association and a Committee of Publishers and Associations

Many of the designations used by manufacturers and sellers to distinguish
their products are claimed as trademarks. Where those designations appear in
this book and Adams Media was aware of a trademark claim, the designations
have been printed with initial capital letters.

This book is available at quantity discounts for bulk purchases.
For information, please call 1-800-872-5627.

Acknowledgments

"There is usually no dreamer so unworldly as the anthologist. He wanders in a vast garden, lost in wonder, unable to decide often between flowers of equal loveliness."

Mary Webb, *The Bookman*

As an anthologist, I have the privilege, and the challenge, of creating creations not of my own creation—of taking the disparate works of many authors and crafting them into a compelling and cohesive whole. My work, then, relies heavily on the contributions and cooperation of many people, only some of whom I am able to acknowledge here.

I am deeply grateful to the authors, most of them nursing professionals, whose stories grace these pages. It takes both courage and skill to tell such personal stories with such honesty, humility, humor, and heart. I am also grateful to the hundreds of writers whose "flowers" I was unable to include in this bouquet.

I would be a ship without a rudder and a sail were it not for the incredible team at Adams Media, who provide an abundance of guidance, support, and friendship. I am especially thankful to Kirsten

Amann, Kate Epstein, Gary Krebs, Kate McBride, Laura M. Daly, Gene Molter, and Paula Munier for all, and I do mean all, that they do.

Thank heaven for Nikk, who has my back and my heart, always. And for my family and friends, who give my life meaning and joy.

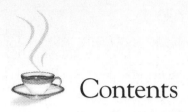

Contents

Introduction ◆ Colleen Sell. vii

Full Circle ◆ Marie Golden Partain 1
Wherefore Art Thou, Julia? ◆ Elizabeth Bussey Sowdal. . . . 8
The Night Al Heel Broke Loose ◆ Elizabeth Turner 13
Something More for Margaret ◆ Shannon Shelton Rulé . . .19
On Borrowed Heritage ◆ Maryellen Clark 26
When the Patient Is Your Mother ◆ Nan B. Clark 32
Of Comrades and Comets ◆ Bonnie Jarvis-Lowe. 39
The Lamplighter ◆ Julie Alvin 45
A Hazard of the Trade ◆ Jane Churchon 50
Inside the Caring Business ◆ Joanna Collie 59
Touched by a Student ◆ Elizabeth-Ellen Hills Clark 67
Aunt Nurse ◆ Cortney Martin 72
Over Coffee with Sister Filje ◆ Nancy Leigh Harless. 78
A Double Dose of Courage ◆ Lyndell King 87
Clarity in the Midst of Chaos ◆ Barbara Brady 92
Full Moon ◆ Linda Lee Hanson 97

The Importance of Being Harold *
    Marilyn J. Hathaway 103

Cloudy with a Chance of Sunshine * Dorothy Wright . . .107

Scared, Healed, Delivered * Shanna Bartlett Groves 114

A Measure of Worth * Donna Surgenor Reames. 119

Do You Believe in Magic? * Shelia Bolt Rudesill 123

Room 108 * Roberta McReynolds 129

Divine Intervention * Joyce Stark 136

My Brother's Keeper * Sandy Keefe 141

Flight of the Gypsy King * Mary Ellen Porrata 146

A Beacon in the Storm * Linda Swann Dumat. 152

On the Other Side of the Bed * Constance R. Shelsky . .157

R$_x$ for the Best Worst Christmas * Mary E. Stassi 163

Lessons from 3-West * Karen Buley 167

My Amazing Shift with the Handsome Dude *
    Kathleen Herzig 174

Hubba Hubba * Kimberly Ripley .181

Specialing Lieutenant Mulkerne *
    Marcella M. O'Malley 186

A Little Love Will Do It * Carol Sharpe 195

Providence * Mary Walsh Morello 203

That Special Touch * Barbara Thatcher 210

Here's Looking at You! * Jenny Lou Jones 214

Nurse Radar * Robin O'Neal Matson. 220

Triumph in Trauma Room One * Sherrie Kulwicki. 230

My First Thank-You * Lucile C. Cason 234

Macgillicuddy * Shelia Bolt Rudesill 240

Lady in Red * Dorothy Wright. 246

Saving Grace * Linda Lee Hanson...................250

You Are the Nurse? * Nancy Leigh Harless...........255

The Stand-In * Elizabeth Atwater 262

A Caring Presence * Elizabeth-Ellen Hills Clark.......267

Zeb and Ruby * Laurel A. Johnson..................272

Relinquishing a Soul * Terry Jean Ratner 278

A Miracle for Miss Mattie * Barbara F. Iffland.........286

The Last Dignity * Lisa Lemming-Morton.............291

The Least of These * Barbara Loftus Boswell 298

The Healing Art of Friendship * Constance L. Gray 301

The Real Virginia * Joyce Franzen Kopecky 307

Tell Your Story in the Next *Cup of Comfort* 310

Contributors.....................................312

About the Editor 323

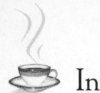

Introduction

"The pitcher cries for water to carry / and a person for work that is real."

Marge Piercy

When I was a tween, in those gangly, wide-eyed years between ten and thirteen, I read, devoured might be a better word, all twenty-seven of the Cherry Ames novels and a few Sue Bartons that I bought for a nickel at a yard sale. In school, I learned about Florence Nightingale, Dorothea Dix, Mary Eliza Mahoney, and Margaret Sanger. Then came the TV series *Julia*, with the title character played by the glamorous Diahann Carroll, and that cinched it: I wanted to be like all of them. (Of course, I also wanted to be like the great ballerina Anna Pavlova and the adventurous writer Willa Cather.) The lives and work of these notable nurses, both famed and fictional, seemed exciting, interesting, and rewarding. If someone would have asked me to jot down a few words describing nurses, I would have said: "brave," "smart," "successful," "compassionate," "noble."

Words like "undervalued," "overworked," "underpaid," and "overwhelmed" would never have crossed my mind. Nor would Jane Churchon's assertion, in the poignant story she contributed to this book, "A Hazard of the Trade," that nurses "straddle the line between the blue and white collars of society." That never occurred to me. Even after the idealism of my youth gave way to the cold, hard reality of the challenges of the nursing profession, I still have always thought of nurses as being in a class by themselves . . . and way up there on the social status ladder.

Of course, I read the newspaper and current events magazines. My best friend, Judy Sebille, a registered nurse, has given me inside glimpses—many frustrating, some inspiring, others humorous—of the nursing world. And I've heard all the stories. At least, I thought I had, until I researched the publications and online bulletin boards of various nursing organizations and then read the more than 800 stories, the vast majority written by nurses, submitted for publication consideration in this book.

What I've learned from the amazing experience of compiling this book is that the nursing profession is even tougher, and richer, than I'd thought. Nurses are, indeed, often overworked and underpaid and sometimes undervalued and overwhelmed. But, as the inspiring stories in *A Cup of Comfort for Nurses* clearly demonstrate, they are also brave, smart, successful, compassionate, and noble. Not to mention dedicated, witty, and wise. But I knew that already. Any profession that can lure my brilliant and fashionable friend Judy away from a successful and lucrative career as a computer scientist and into nursing school in her late thirties and then into orthopedic shoes and a nursing uniform with a stethoscope, rather than a stylish necklace, hanging around her neck has to offer a whole lot more than prestige and a paycheck. Judy is Cherry Ames, Sue Barton, and Julia all rolled into one . . . and then some. She is my hero.

So are the incredible nurses who have cared for my loved ones and me over the years. Like the obstetrics nurse who put a cool washcloth on my forehead and whispered encouraging, soothing words into my terrified ear as a team of doctors and nurses twisted, tugged, and pulled to deliver my breached baby daughter. She was the only medical professional who put her neck on the line by providing a written statement validating my complaints about the obstetrician's negligence in my case. Though I merely filed my complaint with the state medical licensing board and chose not to take legal action, other of the doctor's patients did file malpractice suits, and our combined actions eventually led to the doctor's losing his license.

Words cannot express my gratitude to the nurse at a veteran's hospital near San Diego who convinced the powers that be to bend the rules so that she could wheel my grandfather's deathbed outside so he could see the azure sky and breath in the ocean air he loved so much one more time. A few days later, she called my siblings and me into the ICU; my grandmother and mother had visited with Grandpa the hour before and were in the hospital cafeteria. The nurse explained that my grandfather was trying to decide whether to approve invasive surgery that might prolong his life, though not improve the quality of it. She had given Grandpa a pad of paper and a pen. She had to hold his wrist while he wrote, "What should I do?" We told him we loved him and asked him, "What do *you* want?" He wrote, "No more," and then "Mary?" We promised that we'd take care of his Mary, our Irish-American-princess grandmother. He elected not to have the surgery and died peacefully two weeks later.

I've found that nurses offer comfort and helpful healing tips that no one else can provide. The list of incidents for which I am grateful to good nurses goes on and on.

The point is, most of us on the receiving end of nursing care recognize the sacrifices and contributions that nurses make on our behalf. Though we cannot presume to know what it's like to be in a nurse's shoes, this book is one small way to acknowledge that we do know the value of the person, the professional, who fills them. These inspiring and uplifting true stories, taken primarily from the lives and experiences of nurses, with a few told from the perspective of the patient or the nurses' loved ones, are a tribute to nurses everywhere. I hope you enjoy them.

Colleen Sell

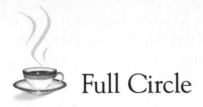

Full Circle

Fear gripped me tightly in its fist as I lay alone in my hospital room the evening before the mastectomy that would give me the chance to live and to enjoy my grandchildren. As an oncology nurse, I was accustomed to being at the bedside of cancer patients, not in the bed as a cancer patient. It was much more difficult than I could have imagined, and in my twenty-three years of nursing, I had never imagined being on the receiving end of my profession. Lying in that hospital bed, feeling more vulnerable and alone than I'd ever felt in my life, I questioned whether the support and compassion that I'd always prided myself on giving my patients had been enough.

My family had wanted to stay longer, but I'd shooed them away, telling them they needed their rest and assuring them I was fine. But I wasn't fine; I was anxious and scared. Then the night-shift nurse came in to give me my pre-op medications. As she adjusted my pillow and lowered my bed to a more comfortable sleeping position, chatting pleasantries to me in a soft, soothing voice, I thought about how kind and how young she was, about the age of my daughter, and how familiar she looked, but I couldn't place her. She was too young to have been on staff when I'd left oncology for psychiatric nursing several years earlier. I assumed she had gone to school with one of my children.

A little while later, the young nurse returned to check on me and to ask whether I needed anything. Though I assured her I was well and didn't need a thing, she somehow saw through my bluff, straight to my fear. I drifted off to sleep with her sitting by my side, her hand resting gently on mine, keeping me silent, reassuring company.

My dreams came easily and vividly that night. Mostly, I dreamt of Paula. I dreamed I was walking on the beach, and I could see Paula and her husband, Shorty, strolling hand in hand on the beach ahead of me, as they had never been able to do.

Twenty years earlier, Paula had been one of my first oncology patients—and the first of my patients to die. Although she ultimately lost her valiant battle with cancer, she had taught me through her example to live each day to its fullest and to savor the simple blessings of life. She was one of the bravest and most beautiful women I've ever known. At the time of her diagnosis, she was twenty-four, married to the love of her life, Shorty, and the devoted mother of their two little girls, ages three and four. She had thick auburn hair that she often wore in a ponytail; that is, until the chemotherapy caused her to lose those luxuriant tresses. Even then, while wearing an elegant scarf or one of her spunky denim hats or absolutely nothing to cover her perfectly shaped bald head, she was still lovely.

Paula's cancer appeared suddenly and advanced quickly. By the time of her diagnosis, it had already metastasized, and aggressive chemotherapy was required to prolong her life. Despite the debilitating effects of the treatments and the relentless onslaught of the illness itself, Paula tried diligently to be a wife and mother, to be actively engaged in her family's lives until she drew her last breath. She was determined to spend every moment she could salvage with her husband and daughters.

There were many complications and setbacks, and Paula was a frequent patient in the hospital where I worked. All the nurses on the oncology unit loved her; there was just something extra special about her. During her numerous hospitalizations, Paula's mother would keep her girls overnight while Shorty slept on the uncomfortable chair-bed in her hospital room.

One of her lowest points was when she was admitted in November, just after Thanksgiving, when her blood platelets and white cell count suddenly dropped dangerously low, side effects of the chemo. The doctors advised that it was unlikely she'd be well enough to return home before Christmas, and she was distressed because she hadn't shopped for Santa Claus for her daughters. The nurses decided we would shop for her. We brought in newspaper ads and catalogs so she could choose what she wanted for each girl, and then we purchased the items and brought them to the hospital. We also brought wrapping paper, bows, and even a small Christmas tree that we helped her decorate. Paula was so happy and grateful to be able to celebrate Christmas with her family, and her little girls were so excited to discover that Santa had delivered their gifts to their mommy's hospital room.

Before Valentine's Day, Paula was well enough to go home—sort of. Because she was still weak and continuing to decline, they stayed at her parents' home, so that her mother could look after Paula and her children while Shorty was at work.

Paula's family had never been to the ocean, and their church had given them an all-expense-paid vacation to a Myrtle Beach resort. Reservations were made for April, and Shorty's boss had given him the time off. In mid-March, Paula contracted a systemic infection and had to be hospitalized. Although she grew weaker by the day, she continued to plan for their much-anticipated vacation.

On April first, I went into her room to check on her, and she beckoned me to her side.

"Call Shorty. Tell him to come now. Mama has the girls, but I don't want them to come," Paula said quietly but firmly. "I don't think I'm going to make it to the beach, Marie. When you go on vacation, please walk on the beach for me."

Although the medical staff saw no physical signs that Paula was nearing death, we had learned in working closely with the terminally ill that often the patient knows more than we do about such things. Shorty rushed to his wife's side. The doctor came immediately from his office to see her and sent her for x-rays. Her lungs were filling with fluid. She wasn't responding to treatment.

Paula and Shorty sat and talked. She dictated letters to both her daughters, which I wrote for her through eyes clouded with tears I could not shed. At shift change that day, Paula left this life she had so loved to be whole and well in eternity. Shorty asked me to stay with her; he didn't want her to be alone, and he had to go break the sad news to his family that Paula was gone. It was Paula's wish that her body not go to the morgue, so I agreed to wait with her in the hospital room until they came to transport her to the funeral home.

I watched through the open door as Shorty, shoulders slumped, walked to the elevator. As he waited for the doors to open, he suddenly turned and came back to the room to kiss his Paula and say goodbye one more time. Then, he started to cry and reached out his arms to me.

"You nurses have been our family for so long," he said as he hugged me. "I'm leaving all my friends. I feel so lost."

I knew we would miss them, too. It was such a difficult time for the family and for those of us who loved them.

That summer, I went to Myrtle Beach and took that walk on the beach for Paula. Just as I've done every year since.

When I was awakened to go to surgery, I was still thinking of Paula. When I was wheeled out of my room for surgery, I kissed my husband and children and tried to be as brave as Paula had always been. The surgery went well, and all the cancerous tissue was removed. Unlike Paula, I had a noninvasive cancer that required only oral medication and regular checkups. Unlike Paula, I am a cancer survivor.

Several months after my surgery, I ran into Paula's mother at the mall. Tearfully, we reminisced, and I told her about my mastectomy and about the young nurse who had been so kind and taken such special care of me the night before my surgery. That's when I learned that the nurse with the familiar face was Paula's oldest daughter, who had been just seven at the time of her mother's death. I also learned that Paula's youngest daughter was currently in nursing school. Paula's mother said that both of her granddaughters had decided to pursue nursing because they remembered all that the oncology nurses had done for their family.

So it seems that compassion, like love, is infinite, an endless circle of giving and receiving that crosses over time and matter, transcending life and death. Just as Paula is with me whenever I walk on the beach in her memory, so too was she with me the night before my surgery, through the presence of her daughter—my nurse.

Marie Golden Partain, R.N.

Wherfore Art Thou, Julia?

When a friend of my daughters' said she was interested in nursing and asked if she could shadow me at work, I was thrilled. As a nurse I'm concerned about the worsening nursing shortage; I'm also expected to do my part to recruit the next generation of nurses. I got permission for her to come to our surgical/trauma intensive care unit (ICU), lent her some cute scrubs, and gave her a solemn lecture on patient confidentiality. Then we hit the ground running. I thought we had a great morning. Nothing too scary happened, nobody pooped while she was there, and we even had time to stop for a doughnut. At eleven, she hugged me, thanked me, and left. *Yay me*, I thought.

Several days later, I asked one of my girls how their friend had liked her taste of the wonderful world of nursing.

"Well, Mom, now she's scared to drive and wants to major in journalism."

Oops.

That made me think. Made me wonder. Where had I goofed? It brought to mind my own early exposure to nursing. Both my grandma and my Aunt Connie were nurses, and I idolized them both. Then, of course, there was Julia.

Aunt Connie was gorgeous and glamorous. She wore pearly pink lipstick and lived in an apartment instead of a boring old house. She even had a roommate who was not her mother or her sister or cousin; she was unrelated and also a very beautiful and glamorous person. They were both nurses. Real nurses.

I knew all about real nurses from watching Diahann Carroll as "Julia" on TV. Nurses were young and fashionable with a strong sense of right and wrong. They had handsome boyfriends who took them out in the evening to places where everyone wore evening gowns and stoles and long white gloves. They lived in fancy apartments, usually in skyscrapers, and everybody loved and admired them. Look at Julia. Look at Aunt Connie.

Though I never actually saw Aunt Connie in elbow-length gloves, she was just the kind of person you would expect to see wearing them. I was pretty sure that Julia and Aunt Connie worked at the same hospital and probably had Cokes and tuna-salad sandwiches and red

Jell-O for lunch together every day. I figured if I ever got to meet Julia, she would love me as much as I loved her and she would reach right into her purse and let me wear some of her Tangerine Tango lipstick.

I was ready for this to happen, because Aunt Connie (The Nurse) had given me a wonderful gift. A real nurse's uniform—crisp and white with a big red cross shining on the pocket right over my heart. And a thing for listening to your heart. And a shot thingy. And a bottle of multicolored candy pills. And a play wristwatch that I wore turned to the inside of my wrist so I would look lovely and graceful when I used it to time stuff. And best of all, most important of all, a real ironing board just my size with a real iron that really got warm so I could keep my uniform looking perfect.

After all that early childhood exposure, it was inevitable that I would eventually become a nurse. Now I am a real nurse too. I have a great big ironing board and a real iron that can really raise a blister if you try to iron before you've had your coffee. I have my very own purse, and I can get into it anytime I want without asking anybody. I own many, many tubes of lipstick, and they all smell nice. That is where the resemblance to my childhood vision of nursing ends.

I have a nursing cap. Somewhere. I even have a picture of me in it, looking like a promo for a questionable B or even C movie. But I have never solved an attempted murder by detecting the subtle aroma of almonds on my patient's breath. In fact, at this point in my career, I have to make a concerted effort and conscious decision to smell anything, having successfully conditioned myself to avoid it for so long. I have never improvised a chest tube from a Giant Pixie Stix straw and duct tape in a convenience store. The words "It will be okay, just give me the gun" have never passed my lips. Well, they have, but only to the bathroom mirror, and I was in my first semester of nursing school, so I think I can be forgiven.

I have never had an ill-fated romance with a dedicated rebel surgeon that ended when he went overseas to save lives. Or any romance with any person medical or otherwise at the hospital. I'm just proud when I remember to say "good morning" to everyone I work with.

No doctor has ever, ever caught me by the shoulders, looked deeply into my warm, compassionate, and yet down-to-earth eyes, and said, "Thanks to you, Nurse, Little Johnny will walk again." Mainly what doctors say to me is, "Where are the graham crackers?" "What was his potassium again?" and "What do you mean, he needs a central line?"

I have learned to ask for a thumbs-up from a patient rather than risk having two or more knuckles broken with a "squeeze my hand." I have had all manner of body fluids, other people's body fluids, splashed, sprayed, and sprinkled on and about my person. I have been called many, many different things, but rarely "Nurse."

I have rolled and repositioned and moved many millions of times my own weight over the years. Just like an ant. I have been scratched, pinched, kicked, glared at, and cursed by crack addicts, bricklayers, and Sunday school teachers. Once, a sweet little old lady tried to strangle me with my own stethoscope.

When I tell my now-retired Aunt Connie about some recent adventure in nursing, she laughs. Laughs! Which tells me that she knew what it was like all along. She knew, and yet she perpetuated the myth. Set me up. Gave me that wonderful white uniform and the iron that got warm, anyway.

So, what do I do when some young woman says to me, "Oh, you're a nurse. Is it hard? Do you like it? I was thinking about being a nurse."

At that moment, I forget what my back feels like, forget that I can no longer wear shorts outside the privacy of my own home for fear my varicose veins will sicken small children, forget the smells and the tears and the stress, and I stand up tall (like someone who might own a pair of evening gloves). Then I say, "Oh, you ought to look into it! It's the best job in the whole world!" And with the wraiths of Julia and Aunt Connie hovering above me, I really, really mean it. It is the best job in the whole world.

Elizabeth Bussey Sowdal, R.N.

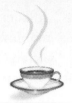

The Night Al Heel
Broke Loose

I n a certain northern city in a certain regional
hospital, a story is still whispered about the
"Legend of Wanda May." It has grown some over the
years, but as one of the few witnesses to the entire
chain of events, I will try to stick to the facts.

Wanda was still a rookie nurse, but a mighty mite
of sorts. Standing 4 feet, 11 inches and weighing no
more than 90 pounds, every bit of her screamed spit-
fire. With her bright green eyes and shiny black hair,
Wanda was a looker. Even the unlikely combination
of a cap that conjured visions of the flying nun and
an oversized scrub suit managed to add to her allure.

Our fifteen-bed intensive care unit (ICU) ran like
organized chaos. With whirring ventilators, beeping
monitors, blaring code-blue sirens, ringing phones,
bright lights, and chatting nurses, sensory overload
was a common problem for our patients. A unique

phenomenon known as "ICU psychosis" afflicts about 10 percent of people treated in this environment. Without warning, a sweet and kindly grandmother can morph into a raving lunatic right before your eyes. With proper medication, the condition usually lasts only twenty-four hours, after which the poor patient is often mortified by his or her earlier behavior.

On the night in question, only three ICU beds were occupied, the first time I'd seen so few patients in our unit, and it was unusually and eerily quiet. As the most senior nurse on duty, I was responsible for responding to and overseeing any codes or emergency situations in the hospital as well as for monitoring the telemetry. I needed to stay at the desk to read the cardiac monitors of both the ICU patients and those in the step-down unit. Phyllis, a jolly and seasoned nurse, was caring for the gentleman recovering from heart surgery and the two-year-old child who had been admitted with severe pneumonia. This left only Alan Heel, who was being looked after by Wanda.

Al was a large fellow with an unruly shock of black hair and an always-ready grin. Looking much older than his twenty-seven years, Al lived a hard life. Severe kidney disease and his penchant for alcohol proved a difficult combination. Weekly renal dialysis had taken its toll, and Al's heart was straining to pump the additional fluids his body could not eliminate. Long estranged from his family, Al was left to fight his demons alone, and his addiction was running amok. He was a frequent visitor to our unit, and we all knew it would be a miracle if he saw thirty.

Al loved the attention he received in the unit, and he was never happier than when Wanda was his nurse. He swore she looked exactly like his favorite stripper, and we would tease and regale him with "Hey Big Spender" whenever Wanda was at his bedside. In spite of all of his shortcomings, Al was easy to like, and we all did.

By midnight of that infamous night, with the patients somewhat settled and the hourly checks completed, we three ICU nurses sat down at the desk for charting and conversation. The unit was shaped in a half circle so that we were in visual range of every patient. Entertaining us with the latest episode of her ill-fated romantic life, Wanda easily held our attention. The reverie, however, was short-lived, as our attention was jolted by the screaming of multiple monitor alarms. In the time it took us to look up, there stood Al, looming over us.

Never have I seen such a sight! Huge and naked except for the monitor leads flapping from his chest, there stood Al, covered with blood. You could have taken his pulse by timing the blood spurting from where he had pulled the arterial line out of his thigh. Blood also dripped from his neck and arm, where his other lines had been only moments before. Despite the blood, the absurdity of Al standing naked in the hall with his catheter and urine bag trailing behind him might have been comical—had it not been for the wild look in his eyes. That glare evoked an altogether different emotion: fear.

In an instant, Wanda and Phyllis were up and on either side of Al, trying to cajole him back to his cubicle, while I grabbed the phone and paged security and then put in a call to Al's doctor. The word "pandemonium" doesn't do justice to the scene that followed. Al Heel had broken loose, and fleeing a demon only he could see, he was running from room to room, dragging his urine bag behind him. Following in hot pursuit were Wanda, Phyllis, two seventy-year-old security guards, and various nurses from the step-down unit. Patients were screaming, the guards were yelling, and the staff was running in all directions. When the on-call doctor and burly police officers arrived, they cornered Al in the hallway, no doubt thinking they had the situation in hand. They didn't anticipate the power of a person, and a very large person at that, in the throes of psychosis. Breaking loose once again, Al ran to the nearest room, a four-bed ward in the step-down unit. The screams of the four elderly female occupants almost drowned out the alarms from their collective heart monitors.

Jumping on top of the nearest bed, Al took a hostage. Now, debate often ensues about the weapon Al used. I hear tell now that it was a butcher's knife, but to the best of my recollection, he had picked up a letter opener from the patient's tray table. Angling the poor woman so that she was perched on top of his naked body, Al held the letter opener to her neck. The frantic look in his eyes gave us all cause to believe that he would use it. Backing off as he demanded, we all tried to think of a way to get a shot of Valium into him. The situation had become truly desperate, and it was at that precise moment that the legend of Wanda May was born.

Extending her arms, palms out to hold us back, she stepped forward. Then, we watched slack-jawed as she flipped off her cap and undid her braid, fluffing her wavy hair. It wasn't until she belted out, in a sultry alto, "The minute you walked in the joint . . . " that I had an inkling of her plan. In front of all of those gathered around the madman marooned on the elderly woman's bed, Wanda began the most raucous striptease imaginable. Her luminous green eyes were focused only on Al. She peeled off her scrub shirt, and as it sailed across the room, Al's wild eyes began to soften. When she shimmied closer, it was plain to see that the occupant in Al's lap hadn't felt that kind of a rise in decades. Once down to her skivvies, with a crooked finger, Wanda beckoned Al to follow.

Like a child in a trance, he put down his weapon and rose from the bed. In utter silence, the assembled onlookers parted, and Wanda, clad only in bra and panties, sashayed through the center followed by Al. She continued humming the strains of "Big Spender" all the way back to the ICU, and patting Al's bed, prompted him to lie down. At that point, I became frightened for Wanda's safety, but instead of venting aggression or sexual energy, Al began to cry. Nestling his head on her chest, Wanda held him, stroking his hair, while the doctor and I started an IV and infused a flurry of drugs. In moments, an exhausted Al drifted off to sleep. Extricating herself from Al's grasp, Wanda casually asked if someone could retrieve her clothes.

Wanda may have been small of stature, but she will forever remain a giant to those of us who continue to whisper her legend.

Elizabeth Turner, R.N.

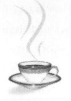

Something More for Margaret

Margaret held the envelopes in her hand. One was large; this would surely be the general equivalency diploma (GED). She could tell by its size. It was thin and flat, and it was addressed to her son. The smaller, letter-sized envelope had her name on it. Her lip quivered, and warm tears filled her eyes. The sound of tires meeting the gravel driveway caused her to look up. It was Arnold, her son. Quickly she wiped away her tears and mustered a smile as he walked toward her.

"Mom, are those the test results?"

"Yes," she answered. She was proud of Arnold. She had homeschooled him since kindergarten and now he was graduating from high school. "Looks like a diploma for you. Why don't you open it?"

As Arnold took the large brown envelope from his mom, he gave a sideways glance at the unopened letter his mother still clutched in her hand. Margaret looked on eagerly while her son tore open the sealed flap and pulled out the diploma. His face looked puzzled.

"Mom, it has your name on it."

"What?"

Arnold handed Margaret the diploma. It was official: There was her name in gold embossed letters. Her eyes lit up momentarily, until she remembered the smaller envelope still in her hand. Then they darkened. She opened the other envelope without a word. It was a letter addressed to Arnold. The labels must have been inadvertently switched on the envelopes.

The letter said that Arnold had done well on the exam, but he had not scored high enough on the essay portion to receive his diploma. He would have to sit again for the essay portion.

"Mom, I'm proud of you. You deserve it," Arnold said. "Don't worry about me. I'll do better next time."

Arnold gave his mother a quick hug and walked inside the house. Margaret stood staring at her diploma. She had passed. Her mind raced with the possibilities.

Margaret had been born into a Mennonite family, and her faith was very important to her. She was schooled through the eighth grade, as was the family custom, and then was sent to Canada to work on an Indian reservation. There, she'd met her husband,

Jim. Several other Mennonite girls were working at the reservation at the time, but Jim was the only Mennonite man. Soon after meeting Margaret, Jim asked her to marry him. Later, after their wedding, they moved to rural Mississippi, where Jim's family lived. Jim found a job, and soon Margaret gave birth to the couple's only child, Arnold.

Like most Mennonite families, Margaret, Jim, and Arnold were very close, and they thrived in their church and community. Margaret taught Arnold with the help of computers and books. She also cleaned houses to earn extra income for the family. She was good at everything she did—raising and schooling Arnold, taking care of her home and husband, cleaning houses, church and community activities—but Margaret wanted something more. As Arnold had grown, a daring new desire had been growing within Margaret.

"You know, Jim," she said quietly one night, "Arnold will be leaving home soon, and I won't be able to clean houses forever. I was thinking maybe I could go back to school."

She watched and waited to see what Jim would say.

"How would we pay for it, Margaret? I'm not against it. I'm just wondering how we would manage."

"I know. I've thought of that. But if this is what I'm supposed to do, then God will make a way."

"Yes, He will," Jim agreed. "What do you want to go to school to study?"

"I want to be a nurse. I think I could do it. I've taken care of people my whole life. I've cleaned their houses; I've tended to the ill and aged. I think I can do it. I think I'd make a good nurse."

As Margaret spoke, the pitch of her voice grew higher and higher with her excitement. It was clear to Jim that this meant a great deal to Margaret, but he had some concerns. They'd manage financially; they'd find a way. It had been a long time since Margaret had been in school, though, and she would need to obtain her GED before she could go to nursing school.

"There would be a lot of sciences," he said.

"I know, but if this is what I'm supposed to do, then I'll be able to do it. I'll work really hard," Margaret said. "It's the first thing I've ever wanted for myself. I want to try."

"Then we'll try," Jim agreed.

Margaret went to the local high school the following week and made arrangements to sit for the same GED exam that Arnold would be taking. (As a homeschooled student, Arnold had to take the exam in order to receive his high school equivalency diploma from the department of education.) If she scored high enough on the test, she would be awarded a scholarship to nursing school. Margaret scored high enough.

She also had to undergo a medical exam and to provide proof that she'd received certain vaccinations. She scheduled an appointment with the family clinic.

"You're here for a school exam?" Dr. McKinley asked. "You're going back to school, at your age?"

"Yes, ma'am."

"My goodness," the doctor said. "What are you planning to study?"

"Nursing," Margaret said. "I want to be a nurse."

The doctor hesitated a moment before wishing Margaret a halfhearted "Good luck."

Luck, Margaret thought, would have nothing to do with it.

For the next two years, Margaret worked hard, harder than anything she had ever worked at in her life. Scrubbing floors was nothing compared to learning anabolic and catabolic cell functions of the human body. Along the way she earned additional scholarships. She went to conferences representing the school nursing program. She joined the nursing club, and sold magazines and made cookies for bake sales, just like the other students.

She rarely saw friends and missed out on many family gatherings and church activities. Both Jim and Arnold supported Margaret every step of the way, taking on extra household duties to protect her studying time. They were not the only ones who looked after

Margaret. A young nursing student named Hettie also took Margaret under her wing.

Margaret looked and acted differently than most of the nursing students in her class. Occasionally there was teasing; sometimes it was hurtful. Hettie would move in and stand beside Margaret, like a silent sentry guarding Margaret from any unkind treatment. Margaret appreciated Hettie's sensitivity, and soon the unlikely pair began to study together. Hettie cheered Margaret, and Margaret encouraged Hettie. Margaret had found a much-needed friend in the younger Hettie.

Margaret successfully completed the nursing program, and two years after receiving her GED, she received another certificate with her name embossed in gold. This one certified that Margaret was a licensed practical nurse. She had done it!

After graduation, Margaret received several job offers. It was no wonder. She'd done exceptionally well in the nursing program and received glowing recommendations from her instructors and advisors. She had considerable experience taking care of people, raising a child, and managing a home, and she had a reputation in the community for being trustworthy and dependable. She had a pleasant and nurturing manner, she loved her work, and as she'd demonstrated through the student nursing program, she was good at it.

Margaret took a job at a medical clinic. When she received her first paycheck, she rushed home to show it to Jim. She would have had to clean several houses to earn that much money. For days Margaret wouldn't cash the check; she just wanted to look at it. Jim laughed with amusement, pride gleaming in his eyes.

Over the next several years, Margaret received job offer after job offer; each new position brought her higher pay and better working conditions. Then one day she got a special job offer that was too good to turn down.

Margaret walked through the employee entrance and put away her things. She washed her hands, straightened her nurse's uniform, and smoothed back her hair. She was ready to report for duty.

She stepped into the hallway and approached the doctor she would be assisting.

"Good morning, Dr. McKinley," Margaret said.

"Hello, Margaret. I'm looking forward to working with you."

"Thank you, ma'am. I'm looking forward to working with you too."

Then Margaret reached for the first patient's chart and walked confidently into the examining room.

Shannon Shelton Rulé

On Borrowed Heritage

Once, Mary Ellen Walton journeyed through the Blue Ridge Mountains on horseback, equipped with nothing but a small satchel of medicinal supplies and the unending compassion that she carried deep into isolated hollows. Today, although my horse runs on six cylinders and gas, rather than on a bucket of oats and apples, I continue her role in the heart of these hills where Appalachian pride still runs deep.

I was not born here; I came here eight years ago, a refugee seeking shelter from the pressures of industrialized medicine. Before long, my hands recognized the taunt of a familiar itch and I scratched it, hoping that I might ease others' pain and offer comfort in time of need.

The shift in my vocational focus brought with it a multitude of impediments. The first obstacle to overcome was fear. I was an outsider, after all, a stranger living among them, and their fear and distrust, while not as predominant as it had been in the past, remained a factor.

Tracking down the location of their homes scattered throughout the county proved to be another difficult task. In the beginning, I spent more time lost than I did found. Hand-drawn maps with notable landmarks scrawled in the margins became my coxswain; their marginal notations held precious tidbits that guided my travels: "Turn left on the dirt road after the sprawling oak that stands alone in the meadow and follow the creek upstream until it forks into twin brooks. Then, take the least traveled path."

No matter where my duties took me, I knew that I would need to take the least traveled path to get there; I always did. Each day began with the knowledge that I would spend the better part of my time sitting one ridge away from where I needed to be, one crest too far to the east, one peak too short of the west. Being in the wrong place was better than being completely lost, but a miss in the mountains leaves you more than a mile off your mark. Eventually, though, I got my bearings and my wheels rolled along dust-laden trails leading to the top of the right ridge.

The leap from an urban career path to a more pastoral one was grueling, and it came with its fair share of stumbles and falls. My ego suffered a few good knocks as I blundered through the transition, feeling as inept as a newbie. In time and with experience, sometimes quite humbling, the bumps in the road eased and the bruises to my ego healed, and my confidence regained its footing—though it wavered on the brink of quitting more than once.

My ignorance of local customs and cultural values created another whole set of challenges. As just one example, it prevented me from recognizing the subtle difference between what folks considered well-intended assistance and outright meddling. And in Appalachia, where no gesture however small goes unnoticed, knowing that boundary is crucial to one's success.

My visits, though habitual, are never routine, and I enjoy the opportunity to meet such diverse needs. I've learned through trial and error, mostly through error, of the unwritten list of "do's" and "don't you dares" involved in providing rural health care, and I wasted no time in committing that list to memory.

I learned, too, that "rooted deep-standing tall" is more than just the county's slogan; it defines the way of life. All one need do is meet one of the elders of the community to see how deep those roots run. Their eyes tell the story: a fierce, inner strength that looked into the bowels of the Great Depression, met it head-on, and won. The old folks spin yarns recounting the skirmishes of more recent battles, too, ones fought with more courage than I possess, waged to defeat a new breed of adversaries—age and the elements. Still, they stand tall. Their integrity and the resoluteness of their self-reliance inspire me. I am enamored of these attributes, I respect them, but most of all, I want them to rub off on me.

It pains me to see the rising sadness on their wrinkled faces as they watch me set an armload of wood by the fire before taking my leave, knowing that I'd just walked that fine line between thoughtfulness and unwanted charity. I learned never to ask first, to just do it. I do what I can to ensure their well-being and comfort, sparing them any prelude or fanfare, leaving their dignity intact. In return, they deliver an unspoken thank-you in the form of a hug. And so the quiet understanding between us has grown.

My calling is not above slopping the family hogs when necessary. Nor has it moved beyond setting a chair near the sink so a woman who lives each day in extreme pain can retain the ability to wash her own dishes, while I dry, giving no mind to how long it might take. Once, I would have struggled against my own impatience, urging me to do it myself in the name of saving time, oblivious to the possibility that, to the client, the simple act of doing dishes might be a saving grace. Now, I look forward to dishpan hands and the passing of time immersed in idle chatter and the latest round of gossip.

In these blue hills of North Carolina, preparing breakfast might involve gathering eggs from a chicken coop rather than a refrigerator. Many a time I have declared through the embarrassment of flushed cheeks that I have no idea how to cook pintos and cornbread, that I have never raised a garden or canned a single vegetable, that I have never tasted, let alone roasted, bear meat, and worst of all, that I cannot make biscuits from scratch. My clients chuckle at my lack of homespun skills and shake their heads, wondering how I have managed to survive all these years without them. I return their laughter and remind them that they're talking to a citified girl who has never made a slice of toast in her life without burning it. Then, I let the amazement in our different upbringings simmer a bit before sharing with them how my city friends always referred to my dinner parties as "BYOF" gatherings—because if they wanted something to eat, they had better bring their own food to the table.

Just as I have taken these mountain folks, one by one, into my heart and under my wing, so too have they found a place for me within their hearts and taken me into their capable hands, teaching me the intricacies and blessings of mountain living. In the process, my hands have served a greater purpose than I have ever known or could have imagined—one that has gone beyond sustaining the quality of life to also sustaining a way of life. Yet, my contributions to their lives seem to pale in comparison to what they have given me in return. Never before have I known such unconditional acceptance, affection, and gratitude, free of judgment, pretense, and reciprocity. Each day spent among these endearing people further affirms my decision to leave facility life behind me.

Mountain health tends many a garden row but none as precious as the spiritual one, the one seeded by symbiotic fellowship that listens beyond the silence and strives to maintain independence—together, as individuals within an integral community. In the evenings, when the dust of dirt roads leaves an inch-thick blanket on the hood of my Tracker and I follow the last ridge home while the day fades softly to night, a deeper understanding of the cycle and miracle of life falls over me. In such peaceful contemplation along these secluded roadsides, I rediscover who I am and why my spirit called me here to serve.

Maryellen Clark, R.N.

When the Patient Is Your Mother

My husband's sister, Emily, met us at the door with her usual confident smile in place, blue eyes calm and knowing.

"Don't worry," she laughed, swinging open the screen door. "Mom's in a really good mood today. She only tried to break my fingers once."

A registered nurse with a degree from Duke University, Emily had specialized in geriatric care in a Connecticut hospital for more than twenty years. Two years ago, after her mother suffered her first mild stroke at the age of eighty-seven, Emily and her husband, Egan, had moved up to Maine and into the old Clark homestead, leaving behind their own newly married daughter without a qualm. Egan, an estate attorney, was able to do the bulk of his work from home. As for Emily, she looked forward to caring for her mother.

"I have three sons, but my daughter is a nurse," Mrs. Clark had often proclaimed proudly. "Certainly no one could have a better retirement plan than that."

After the stroke, she had undergone surgery for several malignant skin lesions. Macular degeneration was destroying her favorite passive pastime, doing the *New York Times* crossword puzzle—in ink. The most worrisome thing, though, was encroaching dementia.

"Might as well see what's up," Tom said, following Emily into the lovely old place with its cozy hooked rugs and comfortable furniture.

"Mom, look who's here," Emily said loudly. "It's Tommy and Nan."

Caught dozing in her old pink wing chair with the newspaper flopped in her lap and her glasses pushed up into her fluffy white hair, she awoke with a start and a frown.

"Bit early, isn't it?" she asked by way of greeting. As she peered at us, the frown deepened. "Getting fat. Both of you. Ugh."

After a detailed explanation of my mother-in-law's bedtime ministrations, medications, morning routine, and dining schedule, Emily took off with Egan to visit their daughter back in Connecticut.

"She can tell if you use milk instead of cream in her potatoes," were Emily's last words to me. "Don't!"

The dinner went smoothly: a meat loaf, fresh carrots, and, of course, mashed potatoes. Standing at the kitchen sink, Tom's mom had grimly scraped with the ancient potato peeler, brown twirls flying everywhere, the rounded chunks, much shaven, gleaming in the water like river stones.

"You're a member of the clean plate club," Tom remarked at the end of the meal as I removed his mother's plate.

"We only say that to children," his mother reproved him.

When I came back with three cups and saucers of old Spode to the heavy mahogany table, Tom was sitting with his hand in his mother's. Wordlessly, she picked it up and started to bend the straightened fingers back toward the knuckles, her eyes riveted on his face. Finally, Tom laughed and broke her grip.

"You're still strong as an ox," he said.

Her face relaxed. "That's what Emily says," she said and picked up her cup.

The weekend went by peacefully enough, and when Emily and Egan returned that Sunday evening, we all had dinner together. Mrs. Clark seemed alert and interested in their adventures, and it was as though old times had returned.

"See, Mom?" Emily laughed. "You're just fine without me."

Her mother frowned. "I am not."

"Mom, you'll live to be a hundred with Emily taking care of you," Tom said.

"That's all?" his mother replied with her old sharpness, and we all laughed.

The next week, however, brought a dramatic shift. Tom answered the telephone on Thursday night to hear Emily's voice, higher than usual.

"It's Mom," she said. "She bit Helen Wilcox today."

"Who's Helen Wilcox?" Tom asked.

"Her hairdresser," Emily said. "It happened so fast, I didn't have time to stop her. We're lucky Mom didn't draw blood."

"For once," Tom joked, but Emily didn't laugh.

My mother-in-law's behavior became more and more unpredictable. At night she'd wander throughout the house, unaware of her own incontinence. During the day she'd fall asleep at a moment's notice, head nodding over a hot meal Emily had just served.

"Em," Tom said in one of the many calls to her, "it's getting to be too much for you. We've got to look at long-care facilities."

"I know what those places are like," Emily said. "And so does she. No way."

The weeks dragged on. Mrs. Clark's condition worsened. Finally, she fell out of bed in the middle of the night and broke a hip. After surgery, she went to rehab in a clean, bright, cheerful place that Emily damned with faint praise, saying, "It's decent, but it's not home."

After almost a month, my mother-in-law did come home. Emily installed an intercom system such as those used to monitor babies. She and Egan had been unable to get a full night's sleep before the broken-hip incident; now they rarely slept more than an hour at a time.

"She doesn't snore exactly," Egan said with what Tom and I thought of as the patience of a saint. "She just breathes loudly enough so you know she's there."

All three brothers and their families went up to Maine for the Christmas holiday, staying in various inns and motels rather than at the Clark homestead to alleviate the burden on Emily and Egan. On Christmas Day, the entire family gathered around the huge oval table in the festively decorated dining room after spending the morning cooking and baking in happy camaraderie while my mother-in-law peeled a mountain of potatoes.

"I want to go home," Mrs. Clark announced suddenly, staring around the table. "Take me home. Now."

"You are home," Emily said. She pushed back her chair and went to her mother's side, bending over her to murmur, "Mom, listen to me. You are home."

Mother and daughter stared at each other. Finally, with a grunt, my mother-in-law tried to push back her chair. "Not the one I'm used to," she said. "You took it."

We all watched as Emily retrieved her mother's walker.

"Come on, Mom," she said. "You'll feel better after your nap."

While the rest of us cleared the table, Emily took care of her mother. When we all adjourned to the living room, Emily reappeared, a strange look on her face.

"Don't anybody say it," she said defiantly. "She just had a senior moment. She'll be fine."

On New Year's Day, Mrs. Clark fell again and ended up in the hospital. Back to rehab she went.

"She can't wait to get home," Emily said every time someone called.

Tom and I drove up from Massachusetts to see his mother on a cold, blustery day with snow in the air. The nursing home's living room was filled with piano music, the scent of cinnamon, and a bevy of white-haired seniors in wheelchairs, but his mother was in her room, her fingers restlessly tearing tiny strips out of the *New York Times*.

"Tell Emily," she said, eyes dropping to her task after looking up briefly, "to sharpen the peeler."

That night, over dinner, Emily's eyes suddenly filled with tears. "I promised her I'd take care of her," she sobbed. "I told her she'd never have to go into a nursing home."

"Times change," Tom said gently. "She's changed. She needs a full-time staff, Em, and you need to cut yourself some slack."

As it turned out, Emily and Egan were there at Mrs. Clark's bedside when she passed away suddenly at four in the morning in the local hospital after suffering a massive heart attack.

"I wish she could have died at home," Emily said wistfully when we arrived a few hours later.

"No way," Tom said firmly. "Even angels can't do it all, Em."

"But that's just it," Egan said, leaning over to wipe away a single tear from Emily's cheek with his thumb. "Nurses always try."

Nan B. Clark

Of Comrades
and Comets

Very few professions foster the kind of close relationships with peers that nursing does. Nurses typically spend more time and have more intensely personal interactions with patients and coworkers than they do with their own families. In the emotionally charged environment of most medical facilities, nursing professionals work side by side, day in and day out, providing care and comfort to sick and dying patients as well as support to their distressed loved ones, inevitably sharing more than just the clinical aspects of the job. As a team, they tackle difficult situations and share their frustrations, losses, and triumphs. To relieve the unrelenting stress of dealing daily with human suffering and myriad other challenges of the profession, such as chronic understaffing and shift work, they talk with and tease one another. And when the pressures of balancing a personal life and a demanding professional life seem like too much to handle, they're there to lend their comrades a helping hand, a shoulder to cry on, or a "you can do it" pep talk.

Not surprisingly, then, nurses often form strong bonds and close friendships with their fellow nurses, many lasting a lifetime. Such was the case for me throughout my thirty-four years in nursing. One of my most memorable and enduring working relationships was with Joy.

For five years, Joy and I worked as R.N.s in the medical unit of a sixty-bed hospital. We were teammates on the same grueling rotation: twelve-hour days one week, twelve-hour nights the next. Whenever a new patient was admitted to our unit, Joy and I always tried to greet the newcomer together. After welcoming the patient by name, I'd announce, "Your nurses this shift are Comfort and Joy." In response to which the patient would either stare at me in bewilderment or ask, "Who did you say was working?" And I'd say, "Comfort and Joy. She's Joy. I'm Comfort." That usually brought a chuckle or a smile to the patient. It didn't take long before the staff started referring to us as Comfort and Joy, too.

Joy was tall, slim, and willowy, with blond hair reaching down to her waist, usually worn in a long braid. I, on the other hand, am dark-haired, fuller figured, and older than Joy by ten years. Joy was timid about expressing her opinion; I was sometimes too opinionated. Joy was born and raised in the town we lived in and her family was a farm family, whereas my background as a Newfoundlander was that of fishing and the sea. Our diverse backgrounds allowed us to teach each other and share the differences between us.

We also shared similarities. Both of us were the oldest of five children; we both had long, stable marriages; we each had children, and those children were a boy and a girl. We lived in a little Nova Scotia village just across the river from the town where our hospital was located. Very rarely did we socialize outside of the workplace, other than at staff parties or hospital functions.

We would laugh at the different lifestyles we lived, and the fact that I could be somewhat of an independent person, enjoying time alone, my family far away in another province, while Joy had her family living all around her on the farmland her family owned. Joy's husband was a professional photographer; mine was in law enforcement. Joy loved china and silver; I love pottery and an out-door lifestyle. Though my children were consider-ably older than Joy's, we had plenty of things to commiserate and celebrate with one another—all of the usual hassles, dreams, joys, and tears of run-ning a household and raising kids, along with the unique impact that our shared profession had on our personal lives. We even sometimes nursed one another through our own illnesses.

Joy and I worked exceptionally well together, and there was never a cross word between us. We knew each other's work habits, and we respected and trusted one another's clinical skill and professional integrity. Together, we made one heck of an efficient nursing tag team. We loved working together, and we loved our work.

But neither of us liked the twelve-hour night shifts. The hours between 7:00 P.M. and 7:00 A.M. seemed to drag on and on. One of our rare breaks from the monotony was an evening maintenance man who, from time to time, would make his rounds on a bicycle, sending us into gales of laughter. One night as Stewart pedaled by on his bike, he mentioned that a comet was visible that night because the sky was exceptionally clear. Joy and I looked at each other with matching expressions of glee and determination. We put our heads together and conspired to slip outside later to search the night sky for the comet. Rounds first, organize the shift, check out the comet: that was our plan.

Around 3:00 A.M., Joy came striding toward me with her cup of tea in hand. "C'mon, let's go gaze at the heavens."

The time was right: The patients were all asleep, the L.P.N.s were there to monitor things, and the sky was still dark and crystal clear. We did a thorough check of the cardiac monitors, took one last glance around the unit to make sure all was well, and left instructions with the L.P.N.s to come fetch us if anything went awry. Then we headed outside.

The hospital was built around a center courtyard, and the first-level walls surrounding the courtyard were made almost entirely of glass. Not far from our nursing station, a set of patio doors opened into the courtyard; from there, Joy and I could look for the comet and still be within sight and shouting range of our unit. A cool August breeze ruffled our hair, and the night sky was magnificent, even without a comet. The twinkling stars looked like a scattering of diamonds against a deep blue velvet background, providing a perfect backdrop for the full moon. It was very still out there, no beepers, phones, buzzers, or alarms to distract us from our astronomical quest. We stood quietly, side by side, gazing upward, occasionally remarking in a whisper about this and that.

Suddenly, Joy pointed upward and said, "Make a wish, Bon."

I looked in the direction she was pointing in time to see a shooting star, which was immediately followed by another and then another one.

Then I spotted it: the comet, bright and beautiful, with its tail a streak of sparkling white light, like something straight out of a movie. We stood in awe, silent, engrossed in our own thoughts as we gazed with wonder at heaven's display, soaking it in. It was a powerful spiritual moment that transcended time and space. Joy and I both felt it, and we were humbled by it.

As we slowly made our way back to our nurses' station, Joy said, "How could anyone see something like that and not believe there is a Power greater than us?" I could only nod in agreement.

We knew how sick some of the people in our care were that night; we knew some of them might not make it to morning. We had needed the spiritual renewal of that celestial moment to help us cope with whatever the rest of the night might bring. Just as we needed the comfort and joy of our friendship to sustain us in our jobs and in our lives.

Bonnie Jarvis-Lowe, R.N. (retired)

The Lamplighter

"Why nursing?" It's a question I've been asked often. Apparently, nursing is one of those professions that those who have no interest in have difficulty understanding why anyone would. For me, the decision to go into nursing wasn't at all difficult to make. My reason and my inspiration for becoming a nurse were, quite simply, my sister Winnie.

Winnie was the fourth of nine surviving children born to my parents. She began her life with severe brain damage and significant cerebral palsy. Believing that she would be more likely to thrive in a loving and stimulating atmosphere, my parents decided not to institutionalize my sister and chose to raise her among their other children in a small four-bedroom house. With no formal nursing training or medical education, my mother became an expert on providing basic nursing care to Winnie.

Winnie's daily routine included spoon-feeding. This involved much time and care because of her difficulty in swallowing and the risk of aspiration. Her immobility and incontinence required meticulous skin care to ward off the constant threat of pressure ulcers. Daily warm baths and massages provided her with much comfort, relaxing her spastic muscles. Cognitively, she was estimated to be at the level of a toddler, and communication was challenging at times. As Winnie got older, she developed frequent grand mal seizures, which necessitated medicating her and keeping her safe when she seized.

Although my mother was Winnie's primary caretaker, my father, my siblings, and I—under Mom's supervision—all participated in her care. Tending to Winnie was an integral part of everyday life in our family. But we never thought of these "nursing" tasks as chores; rather, it was simply the way we lived with, and loved, Winnie.

Winnie lived all forty-four years of her life at home, and she wasn't just kept in the house, hidden from the rest of the world. She was one of us, very much a part of our large, active family. My parents brought her to our school activities and to family outings; she especially loved our regular visits to the park. She went with us to run errands and to visit family and friends. The only place she didn't go with us was to church, out of courtesy to other parishioners, because she would become very loud and disruptive during the service.

Like every member of our family, Winnie had a distinctive personality and made her own special contribution to our family culture. Her sweetness made us smile often, and some of her antics brought on gales of laughter—like when she'd mimic the tone of Dad's voice when he was frustrated with one of us kids. Winnie savored simple things; one of her favorite activities was going for walks outside in her wheelchair. She spoke a few phrases, and one of them was the mournful request, "I want to go out." She had an ornery side, too, and would crawl up to our dog and pull on his tail and not let go. Most of all, Winnie gave us oodles of love, frequently plying us with slobbery wet kisses.

My parents never complained about the amount of care Winnie required or the sacrifices they made on her behalf. They never intimated, or felt, that having a child with such severe disabilities was a burden. Growing up in that environment, my siblings and I naturally adopted similar attitudes and perspectives. As a child I was perplexed when people would remark "how hard this must be" on my parents or us other kids or "how tragic" it was. What they apparently could not see was how "normal" and joyful our home life actually was. In fact, my parents did such a good job of weaving Winnie into the fabric of our lives and ours into hers that it wasn't until I reached adulthood and had a family of my own that I fully realized how amazing what my parents had done was.

As time passed, I and all of my other siblings moved out of our childhood home and went on with our adult lives. As Winnie aged, she became increasingly fragile. My parents, too, got older and developed health problems of their own. Still, they never complained or conveyed in any way how difficult it was to care for her. Though my siblings and I helped when we could, having work responsibilities and families of our own, we were unable to provide regular assistance with Winnie's daily care.

Finally, my parents realized that they needed to have some help in caring for my disabled sister. My sister Katie's family and my family were already living next door to each other when the house on the other side of Katie's home went up for sale. With my siblings' and my encouragement, my parents sold their home of more than twenty-five years and bought the one by Katie and me. Moving out of the home they loved and had raised their children in saddened them, but they were glad that now my sister and I could help provide Winnie with the loving care she had received all her life. The move also gave our children the opportunity to have more firsthand experience with their aunt Winnie.

Five years later, Winnie, at the age of forty-four, passed away from respiratory complications following minor abdominal surgery. My sister never went to school, worked, married, or even had a life outside of our family. At her funeral mass, I wondered how our parish priest would articulate her accomplishments or the significance of her life; certainly, in the conventional sense, her contributions were not obvious. I need not have worried.

The analogy the priest used to describe the impact of Winnie's life was to refer to her as a "lamplighter." Her need for extraordinary care "lit us up" by bringing out the best in us. Her presence in our lives taught us the value of compassion and that life itself is a blessed gift.

Of Winnie's eight brothers and sisters, five of us have chosen nursing as our career. Her radiant light has also spread to the next generation; some of her nieces and nephews have pursued and others hope to pursue nursing and other health-care professions. I work in labor and delivery, and occasionally we care for families who face the challenge of caring for children with lifetime disabilities, and I cannot help but think of these children as future "lamplighters."

Julie Alvin, R.N.C.

A Hazard of the Trade

Leah is a small woman, barely five feet tall, with short, dark, and only slightly thin hair topping an elfin face. She has a confident, matter-of-fact air about her, as if nothing out of the ordinary is really unexpected or insurmountable. Leah is also a miracle.

I am a registered nurse, work that awkwardly straddles the line between the blue and white collars of society. Nurses have a broad base of knowledge and skills. When hospitalized, a patient will see the physician for three minutes a day and three or more nurses several times a day throughout their stay. We are intimately familiar with each patient's disease and its treatment; medications and their effects; and personal preferences in everything from food to the height of their bed, the position of their pillow, room temperature, and TV programming. We clean their vomit, empty their bedpans, and wipe their rear ends. We pull blood from their bodies and put it into their bodies, we interpret the results, and we report what is significant to the doctor. It is important that we know what is significant, and equally important that we let the doctor be the final judge of its significance, in our own finely tuned dance of power with the medical profession. We hold patients' hands, and sometimes we cry when patients can't see us, but rarely when they can.

We are a cynical lot. We've seen too many three-month-olds with inoperable brain cancer, too many middle-aged accountants suddenly felled by a mysteriously burst artery in their heads, too many terminally ill people die, just as predicted. When a patient or friend tells us they have cancer, we begin to silently rate their odds, and we tend to err on the side of doom.

Part of our work is to encourage patients to believe in miracles; on the flip side, we must also help them to accept the inevitable. In a world of complex blood chemistry, chemotherapy, and radiation, we employ words and clichés more at home in a boxing ring than in a hospital. We say, "You can beat it," and "Keep fighting!" We also encourage our patients to "let go" and to know that "we all have only this moment." It is this type of double-speak—the holding of hope in the same breath as the possibility of death—that creates wonderful actresses of most members of the nursing profession.

It is our job to provide these emotional safety nets for our patients and their families. But among ourselves, in the break rooms and locker rooms of America's hospitals, we whisper our truths to each other—that all of us are going to die; that Mr. Smith in 3227 doesn't have a prayer; that those miraculous machines and medicines that are purporting to give life to our patients are truly only sucking the breath and marrow out of some of them, preparing them, even laying the foundation, for death. We stand by, the families stand by, each of us secretly grieving while clouds of hope fly from our mouths, until finally, days or years after the whittling away began, we raise our hands, cry our tears openly, and welcome the glory and the relief of dust and ash.

Two years ago, Leah was diagnosed with multiple myeloma. Yet, here she is, in our living room, her sons playing in our home. Caleb, my son Izzy's best friend, is brilliant, a ten-year-old Einstein. His wire glasses, worn since he was two, sit lopsided on his face, askew and always at the end of his nose, until he distractedly pushes them up, only to have them slide down once more.

Caleb was the first miracle in Leah's family. He was born with hydrocephalus, a condition that would have made him mentally slow were it not for the tube that runs from his skull to his belly, surgically implanted as a newborn. Caleb learned to read at three, can read now at almost college level. The boys attend a Waldorf school, which teaches handcrafts. They used to sit on this couch, knitting, side by side, Caleb a small Harry Potter to Izzy's Alfred E. Newman smile and freckles, the needles *tap-tap-tapping*, the two boys giggling. Over the last year, GameBoys and an Xbox have become the new knitting needles for the pals, the serenading circus sounds surrounding the still-present giggles, as blue-haired Pokémon characters crash magically through massive steel walls.

Caleb's brother, Daniel, is three and a half. Like Caleb, his hair is a thick blond nest, each hair like the tender tendrils that sprout from a carrot, awry and disheveled, not curly, not straight. Daniel wears a blue-and-green striped rugby shirt pulled up to his chest beneath overalls, his sturdy feet in once-white sneakers. Despite his age, he still speaks with a lisp, leaving out verbs and nouns willy-nilly from his sentences, following Caleb through the house. He is unable to either knit or play GameBoy, but he is able to sit, fascinated, in adulation of his older brother.

Today is Izzy's tenth birthday party, and I am watching helplessly as he ceases to be my little boy. He is the youngest child, my last, and only six weeks ago, my own mother died. I am feeling the slipperiness of time, the desire to stop it, freeze it, to somehow hold on to each moment physically with my hands, my body, to keep my son suspended here, free from all the losses and disappointments that are congregating at our door. My daughter, sixteen, is already entering that world of loss. She's found love and lost it again, and experienced her parents' divorce at a time when she was mature enough to see the pain of it. But Izzy is still innocent, for just this moment. Both my parents are dead, and now I'm the grown-up. My urge to protect Izzy grows stronger with each millimeter that he gains, growing away from me and into a mysterious world I still don't understand.

For months before her diagnosis, Leah had an excruciating backache—the symptoms were treated but never dissipated. A trip to an emergency room for severe pain one Sunday afternoon revealed the cause: the myeloma was eating her bones. A simple blood test revealed the cancer. Multiple myeloma is a malignancy of the plasma; first it attacks the blood cells, and then, carried conveniently on the freeway of veins and arteries that line our skin, it spreads throughout the body. It is almost invariably fatal, especially when found late, as in Leah's case. Caleb was seven; Daniel eighteen months. According to statistics, only 3 percent of people who are diagnosed with multiple myeloma in its late stages are expected to live a full year. The myeloma seemed destined to suck Leah away from her own and her children's future, and true to the science I learned in nursing school, I expected a painful death and to see Caleb and Daniel motherless the next spring.

We humans have a mysterious drive to live, no matter what the conditions. We have an unwillingness to lie in defeat, even when defeated. I have seen patients believing until just moments before their deaths that all the conquering and envisioning and fighting would pay off. Leah refused to tell Caleb that she was going to die, a decision that I silently questioned and judged. For almost a year of her illness, Leah was only a faint shadow in her family.

Leah left her marital bed and moved into the downstairs family room, avoiding stairs that were closer to impossible than onerous. She tried to be bright when her boys returned from school, but often fell into exhausted sleep through her days, while her mother, her sister, her friends cared for Caleb and Daniel. Tubes and machines hung and dragged around her as she careened, bald, through the house. She received chemo, and the myeloma spread even further. A round of CT scans revealed a dark mass within her abdomen, close to her liver and pancreas. I heard the bell tolling. Leah had surgery, and the mass turned out to be benign but potentially dangerous if left undiscovered. I believed that she had slithered away from one dark road only to have some other unknown danger lurking, menacing, waiting to *gotcha!* her somewhere down the road, never knowing what or where or when. I was sure that I would see her simply grow thinner, paler, quieter, until the waiting arms of death folded her into their embrace.

Her sister was a match for Leah's bone marrow, and a transplant was done. A bone-marrow transplant is a last effort in the fight against myeloma. It is rarely successful, and in Leah's case, the outcome seemed disappointingly futile. If the transplant was successful, Leah's blood type—not the same as her sister's—should have changed. Instead, it remained stubbornly O positive. Yet, every day Leah got better. Her blood counts began to stabilize. She felt stronger. Once unable to walk more than a few feet at a time, she was able to go upstairs to her own bedroom, leaving the family room to her children again. One day sometime last year, she was simply not ill anymore. She returned to work as an administrator. Leah's last round of tests—blood is gathered and inspected every twelve weeks—came back clean just this week, and now the clock is moving inexorably forward to the next set of tests.

Izzy and Caleb are in Izzy's room, fingers flying on an electronic device, any electronic device. Daniel wanders between Izzy's room and the living room, where the adults are seated, touching his mother's leg for an instant before wandering back to admire his brother.

After about an hour, the almost-four-year-old toddles into the room and announces in a lisping, booming voice, "I pooping."

The two of us laugh, and Leah says with a casual smile to Daniel, "Okay, thanks for telling me," and Daniel wanders away. Leah is wearing jeans and a maroon cotton blouse, with pockets on both sides of her chest. Her shoes are black sneakers, almost orthopedic looking, sensible.

Soon Izzy, dressed in jeans and a now cake-stained green T-shirt, comes into the living room and bites his lip, unusually awkward.

Leah asks him, "Is Daniel stinking up your room?"

Izzy, grinning a sheepish set of teeth. "Uh, well, actually, Daniel does kind of smell. I didn't notice at first," he says, trying to mitigate the bad news.

Leah stands up, thanks Izzy, and the business of changing Daniel's pull-up commences.

She's back a few minutes later.

"A little revenge for being sick?" I ask.

Leah laughs. "Exactly! Let's see, how long was Mommy sick?" She looks playfully at her watch. "A year? Why, that's how long Daniel's going to refuse to get potty trained and how long Caleb will throw temper tantrums over ridiculous things."

"Even miracles have their price," I say.

My mother died of unknown causes at eighty-five. She was suffering and wanted to die. Leah is forty-seven and startlingly alive, despite having a fatal illness. She has a life to lead, children to raise. Sometimes the world is fair and we die of old age. Sometimes the universe does allow us to grasp one more moment, one more ounce of life, or even pounds and pounds of it, against all the odds. Sometimes what we whisper to ourselves, what we nurses and doctors secretly believe of our patients, that there is no hope, that miracles do not occur—sometimes we're just plain wrong. And for now, Caleb and Izzy play innocently in the bedroom, Daniel toddles between rooms, and Leah takes breaths that are mysterious and miraculous gifts.

Jane Churchon, R.N.

Inside the Caring Business

On completing our nursing training, my fellow students and I felt that we were sufficiently prepared to meet any related eventualities with competence and professionalism. However, in later years, working as a charge sister in a small Derbyshire hospital, I often discovered that my qualifications barely equipped me for some of my dealings with the nursing staff and patients on the ward. Indeed, this part of my job simultaneously afforded me my most rewarding and trying experiences. One such memorable occasion took place on a particularly cold and wet day.

Apart from the "live-in" patients on the medical ward, such as Mrs. Hardy with her rather nasty gout and arthritic problems, and sweet old Mrs. KcKinnon with her eccentric cardiac patterns, Whitbridge Hospital was to be graced that day with the admission of a Mr. Franks. His civic prestige far exceeded that of any patient tended thus far in our little hospital. Mr. Franks's imminent arrival had been anticipated with an enthusiasm that hardly befitted his obstructed bowel complaint, but which had, nonetheless, increased staff morale almost to the point of his literally receiving red-carpet treatment. Upon reviewing Mr. Franks's chart, I groaned inwardly to learn that his physician was a certain Dr. Preston, who would be arriving later to see his prestigious patient.

Dr. Preston was renowned for being quick to chide and slow to bless, so to speak. Although not exactly unfriendly, he was a large man and carried such an air of mission that those around him were often propelled into frantic activity so as not to incur his wrath, which, it was rumored, had the ability to reduce a hospital to rubble. Generally, however, he was liked and respected by all, and invariably his visits left some of the younger nurses speechless and blushing in his wake.

Two such nurses joined me on the ward rounds the morning of Mr. Franks's anxiously anticipated arrival: Nurse Cranberry, a mouse of a girl with an ego to match, was a firm favorite with the patients on account of her huge heart and gentleness, and Nurse Powell, who would have been better suited to life within a ballet company than a hospital. With both a passion and a physique for the art of dance, she had earned the nickname "Pirouetting Powell," while making herself unpopular with most of the staff for her aloofness and tendency to rise above her station. Regarding her closely that morning, I wondered what would happen were she and Dr. Preston ever to cross each other's paths.

Coincidentally, it was Nurse Powell who admitted the revered Mr. Franks. I was surprised that such a small man could cause such nervous inhibition among staff and patients alike. His scowl was so firmly in place that it was difficult to decide whether it had been there for years or if it were merely symptomatic of the concentration demanded by his uncomfortable condition.

"Good morning, Mr. Franks," I beamed, determined to change his gray skies to blue. "I'm Sister Blackshaw, and today we're going to make you comfortable and happy so that you're ready for surgery tomorrow. I see you've already met Nurse Powell . . . "

She curtseyed in mock modesty as the spotlight momentarily fell on her. " . . . and if there is anything you need during your visit," I continued, "she will be here to help. We're going to start this morning by setting up a nasogastric tube to assist in draining your stomach, followed by a fleet enema." "I'm having neither," he said in a strained voice.

"I beg your pardon, Mr. Franks, sir. What did you say?"

"I said, I'm not having one of those drain things, and I'm not having an enema, and that's final."

All the diplomacy and persuasion in the world would not make Mr. Franks change his mind. As my cheery demeanor slowly faded to a more menacing stance, Nurse Powell started to *plié* nervously behind the drip, bobbing up and down, ankles together, toes facing outward at opposing angles, back ramrod straight, bending only at the knees as she spoke.

"Sister . . . er . . . Blackshaw, I do believe that Dr. Preston should be consulted for an alternative mode of medical . . . um . . . relief."

"Why, thank you, Nurse. Then I can leave it to you to phone him right away."

Over the phone, Dr. Preston advised me to administer laxative tablets, on account of the acuteness of the patient's condition, and, I fancied, as a defiant gesture to Mr. Franks's stubbornness. After jotting down the order, I gave it, along with verbal instructions, to Nurse Powell as she floated past me in the hall.

"Yes, yes. I myself would have advised as such. Do not fear, Sister . . . Sister . . . what is it? . . . Blackshaw. Yes, of course. Leave it to me."

I'll leave your wonderful Dr. Preston to you, too, I thought grimly.

Sitting with a cup of coffee at lunchtime, I began to feel better about the doctor's impending visit.

After all, the medication had been administered, and tomorrow the little man would be off my ward.

It was 1:30 P.M. when Nurse Powell first deigned to seek my aid.

"Sister . . . Blackshaw, I gave the fourteen laxative tablets to the patient, but I'm sorry to report that Mr. Franks has had no, er, bowel movement. He has, however, been vomiting continuously since eleven o'clock."

"How many tablets, Nurse?"

"Fourteen, Sister, as you said."

"I told you to give him four tablets. I even wrote it down."

"Fourteen, Sister, you wrote 'fourteen.' I have the paper." She rather ungracefully ransacked her uniform pockets before retrieving the note. "Oh . . . um . . . I see now that you, indeed, wrote 'four.'"

With all dignity stripped away, Pirouetting Powell was at last reduced to the trembling form of the dying swan.

"Please don't tell Dr. Preston! Whatever shall I do?"

Leaving her to face her final curtain in privacy, I dashed into Mr. Franks's ward, wondering what scene of destruction awaited me. However, apart from looking pale and a little self-absorbed, Mr. Franks looked surprisingly controlled.

I swallowed, took in a deep breath, and smiled winningly. "And how are you feeling, Mr. Franks?"

"I'm not having an enema, and that's final!" he barked.

As the man's scowl deepened and his nostrils twitched in anger, I realized that our Mr. Franks was made of firmer stuff—of a sort capable of giving fourteen of the strongest laxatives on the market a run for their money. Nurse Powell, on the other hand, was visibly wilting, and certainly, over the next three hours, she suffered excruciatingly on Mr. Franks's behalf. I could not understand how a professional nurse could be so stupid. Precisely what the patient's condition would be on Dr. Preston's arrival was anybody's guess—if the doctor had a patient at all by then.

I visited Mr. Franks three times as we awaited Dr. Preston that afternoon. He soon ceased all efforts at communication. With eyes bulging, nostrils flaring, and ribcage heaving arrhythmically, the little chap heroically focused all of his attention on fighting the battle raging within.

It was with the patient thus preoccupied that Dr. Preston swept into the ward at 4:45 P.M.

Slapping his hands on the end of the bed, the doctor glared at Mr. Franks's face.

"How are you, Mr. Franks?"

There was no reply, but the livid, unmistakable challenge that had returned to Mr. Franks's expression seemed, mercifully, to satisfy the doctor.

"Did he take the medication, Sister?"

"Yes . . . yes, doctor. He most certainly did."

My desire to get away from the scene of imminent explosion, either on Dr. Preston's part or that of the patient, was almost overwhelming. Nurse Powell, the traitor, had long since disappeared. As the seconds slowly ticked by, I nervously watched as Dr. Preston, plunging his hands into his pockets, grunted thoughtfully and approached Mr. Franks's head. My pulse stopped as the doctor, pausing only a moment, brusquely brought his face to within centimeters of the patient's and stared intently into it. No words were needed as the patient's eyes shot undiluted fury into the doctor's own.

Straightening, Dr. Preston inhaled deeply before turning on his heel and striding toward the door.

"Sister, keep me informed of his progress," came the command.

Within seconds, the whirlwind was gone. Leaning against the wall outside Mr. Franks's room, I thought I saw a tall, slim shadow dance daintily out of sight.

I spent the remaining twenty minutes of my shift preparing the other patients' medications. I admit that I avoided Mr. Franks's bed as much as possible, praying constantly that I would be spared the horror of witnessing the inevitable devastating effects of the medication. At precisely 5:30 P.M., as I prepared to make my escape, I saw Nurse Powell for the first time since Dr. Preston's visit. Her lower lip quivered while her eyes locked with mine for an instant, before she scuttled away to the safety of the ward. I looked forward to a quiet evening contemplating how I could assist in shaping her future: She certainly deserved disciplining, but I knew that the most important lesson had already been learned; perhaps she had received punishment enough, I reasoned.

From that day forward, I never had difficulty in my working relations with Pirouetting Powell. She conducted herself with a modesty far more befitting her position and awarded me the respect mine deserved; moreover, she never again forgot my name.

As for poor Mr. Franks, his time of suffering was mercifully ended by a visit to the bathroom—the duration of which, I heard, continued long after I left the ward.

Joanna Collie, as told by Sr. Blackshaw, R.N.

A version of this story was first published as "The Bottom Line," in *Personality* magazine, November 26, 1993, South Africa.

Touched by a Student

As a nursing instructor, I am charged with teaching my students both the science and the art of nursing. That means not only conveying the technical and practical aspects of nursing, but also inspiring them to apply that knowledge and skill with passion and compassion. Sometimes, however, it is the student who instructs and inspires the teacher. This was true of Dolores.

Dolores was an older, nontraditional student in my clinical group, who traveled a long distance to campus with her best friend, Alison. Though I'd never before had Dolores as my student, I knew through other students that she had a history of cancer that was in remission.

After semester break, Alison asked to speak with me privately. She related that, over the Christmas holiday, Dolores had undergone major surgery to treat a recurrence of her cancer. The surgery had not gone well, and Dolores's prognosis was poor. Her cancer had metastasized, and the surgical site was not healing well. There were few options for further treatment. Dolores wanted to finish her last semester of nursing school, but Alison wasn't sure whether she could, or that she should. She wondered whether Dolores was in denial about the gravity of her condition. She was concerned that going to school while helping her husband to raise their four teenage children and undergoing chemotherapy might prove too much for Dolores. She feared the loss of her friend. She asked me to speak to Dolores, and to encourage her to drop out of school so that she could take care of herself.

I, too, wondered whether Dolores was making the right choice. *Nursing education is rigorous; will it be too stressful and physically taxing for her? Is she setting herself up for failure? What if the chemotherapy fails to arrest the cancer; if she has only a few more months to live, shouldn't she spend as much of that time as possible with her family and enjoying life? Isn't it more important that she take care of herself than other people?* After much agonizing thought, I decided that Dolores must answer those questions for herself.

I also decided to apprise one of my colleagues of the situation, in part because I needed her moral support. More important, though, I felt it was prudent to inform someone in authority that a seriously ill student would be present, in the event any issues might arise related to the student's illness or performance. I spoke with the director of nursing at the hospital where Dolores would be completing her clinical rotation. I explained that one of my students had cancer and might become quite ill during the rotation. I didn't identify who the student was. I would do that later, when and if the need arose.

During that semester, every student missed some clinical time—except one, Dolores. She had scheduled her chemotherapy treatments for Thursdays so she would have the weekend to recover. She didn't want to miss any class or clinical time. During that semester, students complained about many things: their workload, the faculty, unpleasant people and situations in their clinical rotations, their spouses and children, personal responsibilities, and other stressors in their lives. Dolores never complained about anything. She arrived each day with a positive attitude and sought learning at every opportunity. She gave support to her peers and compassionate care to patients. She never asked for an extension on her paperwork, for a makeup exam, or for any other special favors. She never mentioned her cancer directly.

One day Dolores arrived at postconference laughing with delight. A patient had complimented her on her beautiful hair, not realizing that it was a wig covering her bald head. Another time she talked about her need to finish the nursing program. She had once believed that she wasn't smart enough to go to college, and now she was proud of her accomplishments. It was her dream to become a nurse, and she was determined to realize that dream. She wanted to be a role model for her teenage children. She wanted them to be proud of her.

As Dolores spoke, I realized how flawed my thinking had been. She was not ignoring her illness or in denial about her approaching death. She was embracing her life. She wasn't depriving her children of the benefit of her remaining time. She was showing them how to live. She was sharing the importance of setting and achieving goals. She was conveying how much she valued her education. She was demonstrating courage, perseverance, and the importance of living life to its fullest. Dolores was a wife, a mother, a friend, and a nurse, and she found joy in each of these roles.

At our final evaluation conference after graduation, the director of nursing asked me, "You know the student with cancer you spoke of? I kept trying to figure out which one she was, but I never did. So, who is it?"

I smiled and said, "If you couldn't tell, perhaps you weren't meant to know." I thought that was how Dolores would have wanted it.

Dolores died a few months after her graduation from nursing school, but it isn't her death I remember, it is her life. As a nursing instructor, I am fortunate to witness the transformation that occurs as a student grows from novice to professional nurse. Dolores's life serves as a constant reminder of the importance of that process—that the journey is as important as the goal. Sometimes, when I am stressed or dealing with a particularly frustrating student, I hear Dolores's laughter, think of her courage, and remember her determination to persevere. Through the indelible inspiration she left with me, Dolores has touched the life of every student I have mentored in his or her journey to become a nurse. Through that legacy, Dolores—the nurse, the teacher—lives on.

Elizabeth-Ellen Hills Clark, R.N.

Aunt Nurse

When Karen was eight years old, she went to the hospital to undergo surgery for a weak heart. Everything was bright white and cold and seemed to move very fast—like how she imagined the tunnel on the way to Heaven would be. It was the scariest, strangest place she had ever seen. It was only natural for Karen to associate the hospital with things ending. After all, that's where her grandmother had been before she "passed" and was buried in the ground. It was where her kindergarten teacher was when the class found out she had something called "cancer" and wouldn't be back to teach them.

The doctors talked in words Karen didn't understand, in a secret language only grownups knew. They said things like "heart murmur" and "EKG," while her parents nodded with blank expressions on their faces. Then Karen heard a word she recognized: "surgery."

Her parents told her to be brave. They said the surgery would happen while she was asleep and she wouldn't feel a thing. They reassured her they'd be right there when she woke up, that everything was going to be just fine. But Karen didn't feel fine; she felt worried. Scary thoughts filled her mind: *What if she never woke up? What if she never saw her parents or friends at school again? What if she got buried in the ground?*

She trembled when the anesthesiologist came into the room. As he started the medication, Karen noticed the surgeon consulting the operating staff nearby and that the room felt even colder than before. She wondered whether her heart was still beating, and then everything faded away.

When Karen opened her eyes, a woman in white was humming as she straightened up the room. No one else was around, and the harsh light made everything look fuzzy. It was a new room, different from the one where she'd had surgery. Karen wondered if it was Heaven.

"Hi, there," the woman in white said in a tone as soothing as hot chocolate in winter. "How are you feeling?"

Karen was silent until her eyes adjusted to the light and she could make out the woman's features. She had a glowing smile and big, sweet cow eyes.

"Okay," Karen said, though she wasn't quite sure how she felt. She was still trying to make sense of what had happened while she was asleep and what was happening now.

"Are you an angel?" Karen asked.

The woman's laugh tumbled gently off her lips. "No, sweetie. I'm your nurse," she said, emphasizing the word "nurse" as if she was proud of it. "I'm here to take care of you."

Karen liked that idea. She felt more relaxed than she had since she'd arrived at the hospital.

The nurse offered her puzzles and books. She explained what she was doing as she took care of Karen, and she warned her whenever something was going to hurt or feel uncomfortable. When there was nothing to say, her nurse just hummed a sweet-sounding tune that made Karen forget how bad her heart felt.

Over the next few days, Karen watched with wonder as the woman in white with the gentle cow eyes and wide smile tended to her and the other patients. She decided that the nurse must be very kind and strong to take such good care of people who were so sick and in so much pain.

"Miss Nurse," Karen called one day when the pain of her surgery was all but forgotten. "Will I get to go home today?"

"It looks like you will, my dear."

Karen felt relieved. "And you don't have to call me 'miss,'" the nurse added. "You can save that for your teacher at school." She smiled wide and tapped Karen on the nose.

Karen smiled too but didn't say anything back. She was too shy to ask her nurse's name.

Later that morning, Karen's parents came and loaded all the balloons, flowers, and toys into the car. Karen changed from her hospital gown into her clothes and climbed into the wheelchair for the ride to her parents' car. That's when she got a little nervous, because as much as she wanted to go home, she also wanted to say goodbye to her special nurse. Just then, Karen caught sight of her in the hallway.

"Miss Nurse!" she yelled.

Her nurse turned around and smiled. "Now what did I tell you about that 'miss' business? You and I are old friends by now, Karen," she said, squatting to the little girl's eye level and nudging her lightly on the arm.

Karen reached out to give her a hug. "I'm going to miss you . . . ," she thought for a moment before adding, " . . . Aunt Nurse."

When Karen pulled away, she noticed that her nurse's nose and eyes were red and that tears streaked her smiling, glowing face.

"I'll miss you too, Karen."

The image of her special nurse, smiling and crying at the same time, remained etched in Karen's mind long after she left the hospital. In fact, it stayed with her long after she grew up and even when she next entered a hospital—that time, by her own choice . . . as a nurse.

Karen worked as an R.N. in the cardiovascular program of a community hospital, much like the one she had spent time in as a child. Karen's patients were her life. Although she never told anyone, they were what kept her spirits up through an agonizing divorce and the deaths of her parents. They were what steadied her when she felt nervous about her children starting school, going on first dates, and learning to drive. Through all the curves and challenges and changes that life brought over the years, Karen's relationship with her patients remained a constant source of comfort to her. All of those people lying in hospital beds recovering from open-heart surgery might not have realized it, but Karen needed them as much as they needed her.

Karen sometimes told her patients about her own childhood heart surgery and the "Aunt Nurse" who had been so kind to her and inspired her to be a nurse. She found that it made them feel better knowing she had once been in their shoes.

"That's amazing," said one patient, a forty-something minister named Gary, after she had told him the story.

"Oh, not really." Karen shrugged it off. "Lots of children have surgery to repair defective hearts."

"I'm sure they do, but that's not what I meant," Gary said. "What I meant was that it's amazing how life imitates life. It must be so gratifying to you to know that your patients feel the same way about you that you felt about your 'Aunt Nurse.'"

Karen was caught off-guard; she hadn't ever thought about it that way.

Gary continued, "I've been here a day, and everybody wants me to be strong so they can be strong. But to be honest with you, it's scary.

"And then I think of you. I can't imagine anyone being stronger than nurses like you, who do what you do. You're here every day; you've seen people walk out of here healthy, and you've seen people die. . . . "

Karen nodded, silently acknowledging the sad reality of the lives she had seen lost on the operating table.

"Since I've been here, you've made me feel like I'm the most important patient in the world," Gary said. "But I suspect that, really, you're everyone's 'Aunt Nurse.'"

Karen felt a tear forming in the corner of her right eye. She resisted the urge to suppress it and let it fall recklessly down her cheek. It was very humbling to finally understand what her Aunt Nurse must have felt when Karen had hugged her goodbye.

As Karen left Gary's room to check on her next patient, she took a moment to reflect on what he had said. She smiled. She glowed. Her heart felt stronger than ever.

Cortney Martin

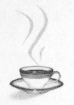

Over Coffee with Sister Filje

"I do not know what they think of me. I think they wonder what kind of woman works so late in the night wearing only her pajamas," the delightful nun told us with a wink.

This feisty little Albanian nun is also a nurse. She was the entire health-care system for her village. Her name is Sister Filje.

I was in Kosovo working in the war recovery effort. A nurse practitioner, I trained local nurses and doctors to provide prenatal care in remote villages six days a week. On Sundays we rested. One Sunday, my friend and driver, Salami, offered to take me to mass in a nearby village. That's how I met Sister Filje, in the mountain village of Latnice, in the former Yugoslavia, an old country with many new names. Red tiled roofs of the villagers' homes dotted the mountainside. In the valley below stood a simple, yet beautiful, 400-year-old church with a tall, stark steeple that soared toward the sky. Next to the church was a small, plainly furnished clinic.

Sister Filje proudly invited us in to see her clinic, and proud she had reason to be. Unlike the filthy, government-run *ambulantas* I had been working in, where we might have to run a rodent out in the morning or at the very least clean up their droppings from the floor, Sister Filje's clinic was spotless. Sparkling glass containers holding small amounts of gauze, cotton balls, and tongue depressors lined the countertops. The exam table, a worn leather-covered cot, was draped in a lovely, pristine-white crocheted tablecloth. A tiny embroidered pillow lay on it, ready to cradle her next patient's head.

When I met her, Sister Filje was probably no more than thirty-five years old. Slightly built, her traditional nun's dress seemed to almost swallow her up, and her dark brown hair peeked out from under her habit. Her kind brown eyes were luminous and expressive, and a dimple in her right cheek appeared and disappeared as she spoke.

She had been stationed in the village for fourteen years, her tenure spanning both before and during the recent war. Despite the incredible amount of misery she had seen in her life, she had a resiliency that belied her petite size and maintained a positive attitude and a delightful sense of humor.

Sister Filje spoke only Albanian. I speak only English. After introducing us to each other, Salami translated that she was inviting us for coffee. Nothing happens in Kosovo before coffee, or more aptly put, everything happens over coffee. This is a significant custom, and no matter where you are, in a home, a school, or a hospital, you are offered Turkish coffee. It is the polite thing to do. It is also the polite thing to accept. To decline is unthinkable. Soon we were balancing miniature cups on child-size saucers and stirring them with tiny spoons. As I sipped the thick black sludge, flashbacks of childhood tea parties involving mud tea danced through my head.

I was interested in her work. As we visited, I asked Sister Filje to describe a typical day in her clinic.

"Yesterday," she replied, "I treated all six of the Rexhepi children for chicken pox. Then I cleaned the earwax from an old man's ears so he could hear just a little of today's mass. Later in the afternoon I sewed a long cut in a young man's leg—he'd gashed it with a sharp hand tool. I see many such cuts now that the tractors are gone. Our men work only with hand tools now."

Her comment about the tractors reminded me how hard life is for the Kosovo farmers since all farm equipment was confiscated by the military during the war.

Sister Filje told me that her work involved not only providing medical care for her patients but also providing social services in the village. Sometimes that meant cooking soup and delivering it to patients who were ill. Sometimes, when the day-to-day stresses of living began to fray the fabric of a family, she was there to offer counseling. Sometimes she got to distribute clothing donated by an American church to the village's children.

"Now, that is a fun thing to do." She winked.

She provided complete, holistic care for her village, but the one thing she didn't like to do was deliver babies. She found that responsibility simply too frightening. When possible, she preferred to transport a laboring patient to the nearest "health house" rather than deliver her at home or in the village clinic.

As we sipped the cups of pungent coffee sludge, Salami and I listened to Sister Filje describe her day. It was obvious that this was much more than simply her work. It was her mission.

I asked her to tell me some of her most interesting nursing experiences in Latnice. Bear in mind that my translator, Salami, speaks Albanian very well but only a little English. I am certain much was lost in the translation, but as I understood it, this is what Sister Filje told us. . . .

A young woman came to the clinic late one night in labor.

"I was familiar with this patient. I knew she was pregnant, and I knew the woman was not normal," Sister told us.

This could be interpreted that the woman was mentally ill or developmentally delayed, or perhaps she meant that the pregnancy had not progressed normally. I was unclear on the details, but this much I did understand: The woman was in active labor, and for Sister Filje, "Delivering babies gives me too much fright!"

So, even though the Sister had already dressed for bed, she quickly loaded the woman into her beat-up little beige Yugo and sped off into the night, bumping down the rut-filled road with the laboring woman screaming loudly in both fear and pain.

"I was terrified. I prayed hard for the baby not to come," Sister Filje said, as she relived the story for us. "She screamed so loud, I thought, 'The health house is too far away; I will drive to the soldiers' base, and the doctors there will help us because this is an emergency.'

"But, they said, 'No. Drive on to Viti to the health house. This woman is Albanian. We can only serve Serbians. The doctor in Viti will deliver her baby.'"

Frustrated and frightened, Sister Filje sped off again into the night, completely convinced the baby would come before they reached the health house. As she told the story, she patted her chest quickly in pantomime of her racing heartbeat, and her eyes were wide with fright. Yet, the mischief still danced in her dark brown eyes, and the dimple in her cheek winked at me.

They did arrive in Viti before the baby was born, and she was delivered safely, mere minutes after they arrived. The infant girl was named Christine in honor of the nun. It was only after mother and newborn were settled into bed for the night that Sister Filje realized she was standing in the health house clad only in her pajamas. She blushed with embarrassment and quickly departed, retracing her path home along the dark, bumpy road.

A few minutes after leaving the health house, she remembered the curfew. In all the excitement, she had completely forgotten that a nine o'clock curfew had been set by the government and was being firmly enforced by the peacekeeping forces. Violators were being incarcerated.

At the military checkpoint she was stopped and made to get out of her car by two machine gun–toting young men dressed in drab army green. They inspected her car and interrogated the little nun. She was mortified as she stood before the guards in the bright beam of their flashlights wearing only her thin blue pajamas. Blushing bright red, she tried to explain why she was out so late in the night and why she wasn't properly dressed.

"I do not know what they thought of me. Perhaps they wondered what kind of woman works so late in the night wearing only her pajamas, eh?" she joked. "And I think they did not believe that I am 'Sister' Filje," she said with a wink and, once again, that sweet dimple. She pantomimed being handcuffed by crossing her wrists.

"They arrested you?" I asked incredulously.

Sister Filje laughed. "Yo, yo, yo," she said.

Even I could translate that meant, "No, no, no."

We all shared a hearty laugh over the image of the little nun standing outdoors in her pajamas trying to convince the soldiers what had just happened.

This is one amazing woman, I thought as I took another sip of bitter coffee. It caused a spasm in the back of my throat, but I just smiled and swallowed, knowing that was the only polite thing to do.

I asked her to tell me about the most complicated patient she had ever treated.

"In my ambulanta, God made a miracle," she said solemnly.

She went on to explain that an elderly woman had come to her with a huge lump in her breast. Sister Filje tried to get help from the nearby military base's medical facility. Solders from several countries were stationed in Kosovo as peacekeepers, and these allied forces maintained a modern clinic and a small hospital near Sister Filje's village. The soldiers, however, turned the nun and the old woman away at the gate. They told Sister Filje to take the woman to the large government hospital in Pristina, more than three hours away by car.

The hospital in Pristina would certainly have treated the woman, had Sister Filje been able to get her there. But convincing her to ride in a car for the ten-minute drive from the village to the military base had been difficult enough. Until that day, the elderly woman had never left her village or ridden in a car. The idea of riding in a car to "the big city" was simply more than she could handle. She adamantly refused.

"Take me home," she told the nun. "I want to die in my village."

"What was I to do?" Sister Filje asked with a mischievous smile lighting her face and making that dimple wink again. "So, we returned to my ambulanta, and I did the surgery myself. No anesthesia! I cut out the cancer, and then I gave her all the antibiotics on my shelf. Now, thank you God, she is well. No infection. No carcinoma. God did a miracle in my clinic!"

Our cups were empty, save for the finely ground sediment that remained in the bottom, and it was time for us to go. The morning had flown by, and I wished for more time with Sister Filje, more time to hear stories over miniature cups of thick, dark coffee, but we all had obligations and so our visit was concluded.

A few days later I left Kosovo and returned to my Midwestern home. Once there, I told this story to many of my colleagues in the medical field. Most of their replies went along the lines of an incredulous, "Humph, it was probably just an abscess," to the more sympathetic, "A benign breast lump, maybe?" Certainly, as professionals in one of the most technologically advanced medical systems in the world, their skepticism is understandable. But then, they didn't meet the remarkable little nun with the luminous brown eyes and the dimple in her cheek that winked as she told her stories. I did, and I choose to believe the miracle version. Now you can decide for yourself.

Nancy Leigh Harless, C.N.P.

A Double Dose
of Courage

I was seventeen, a recent high school grad with six weeks of preliminary nursing training under my belt. Six weeks is just enough time to learn you don't know squat. Every morning I put on my horrid starched nursing cap and looked at the impostor in the mirror. I didn't feel like a healer. I walked onto the ward with my new shoes squeaking softly on the polished linoleum, trembling so hard I thought my knees were clicking a rhythm, my fingernails digging into the palms of my hands with fear that someone might ask me to do something I wasn't prepared for. Sick people often need things—now—and if you're the only one there, you're the one—ready or not—who has to do what they require.

I could have relaxed. The trained sisters watched us like hawks. The patients on our female surgical ward were in good hands. And we nurse trainees were assigned only safe and simple tasks, such as giving sponge baths, making beds, and if we were lucky, taking temperatures.

About eleven o'clock on what had been a fairly routine (though rather nerve-wracking) morning, after I'd finished most of my sponge baths and was about to go for my morning cup of tea, a local farm woman was admitted to our ward. Her hubby had been trying to fix their tractor, and had left it idling while he tinkered with the engine. Big mistake. It was an old piece of machinery. The engine's vibration shook the transmission into gear, and before anyone was the wiser, the tractor took off down the hill on its own. The farmer tried to jump on board to stop it, hollering like a banshee at an Irish wake, trying to alert anyone and anything in its path, but to no avail. Our new admission was milking their cow when the tractor came barreling down the hill, ploughed her under the beast, and amputated both of her legs. I don't know how the cow fared.

The woman suffered through a nightmare ambulance ride with sirens wailing, a swift pass through the emergency department, several hours on the surgeon's table, and a few hours in post-op recovery. Now she was being shuffled off the gurney onto a hard hospital bed on our ward—her two bandaged stumps providing horrifying evidence of her ordeal—while I stood by, bug-eyed, holding a spare blanket from the warming cupboard. If ever there was a nursing situation beyond my expertise, this was it. The sister in charge shooed me off for my tea break. It took me a few seconds to leave, preoccupied as I was with trying to imagine what the poor farm woman was going through.

Half an hour later, I returned to my work covering the end of the ward, which basically meant I poured drinks, fetched and emptied pans, and called for one of the sisters if anything else was needed. I poked my nose into the amputee's room. She was a tiny woman, even smaller now with a large part of her removed. She'd lost a lot of blood. Her face was so white it blended with the sheets. She sat, semireclined in bed, propped up with pillows, a Bible resting on top of the blankets. Her hands clenched it open, fingertips blanched from the pressure of her grip. I figured she was in pain. Swallowing my fear, I stepped into the room.

"Do you need more morphine?" I offered.

She shook her head. Her eyes, shiny with unshed tears, never left the open page of her Bible. I wondered how she managed to read. Though I was not brought up in a Christian household, I was glad she had a faith to hold on to. It seemed to me she was going to need it; her life had undergone a drastic, irreversible change.

"Can I fix your pillows or get you a drink?" It was pathetically small comfort to offer in the circumstances, but it was all I had.

I stood there, quiet, waiting for her response, trying not to fidget, not knowing whether to go or stay. I so wanted her to know how sorry I was that this had happened to her, but I didn't know how to say it. Then, she looked up at me, and her blue eyes seemed to gaze into my soul. She gave me a small, wavering smile.

I've never known anyone braver in my life, I thought.

"Is there anything I can do for you?" I offered. I had no clue what that might be, I just knew I desperately wanted to do something, anything, to ease her misery. It's awful to see someone in pain and not be able to fix it.

"Yes, dear," she said sweetly. She patted my hand. "I hate to ask, only . . . ."

I leaned forward, willing her to tell me what I could do, how I might help.

"My husband, he's outside in the waiting room. Could you comfort him? He blames himself. Would you let him know I'm all right? Tell him it's not his fault."

Have you ever had someone kick a soccer ball, hard, into your gut? That's how I felt at that moment. I could hardly breathe from the impact of her request.

The lump in my throat was so big I could barely swallow. Not daring to speak, certain my voice would crack, I nodded my head and fled the room.

I took a cup of tea and a heart full of sympathy to the amputee's husband. He sat in a hard plastic chair in the visitor's lounge, shaking wretchedly, his face buried in his hands. While I put my teenage arm around him as he cried like a baby, something inside me changed irrevocably.

What comfort I provided the farmer and his wife paled in comparison to the gift I received. That day, I discovered what heroism is. It's not the big tough guy in the movies or comics who battles imaginary forces of evil and conquers the world. A real hero is a little, sick woman, in real pain, looking down the barrel of a changed life and years of rehabilitation, who saw the need of a man for forgiveness and the need of a young nurse for purpose. Even Hercules didn't show that kind of strength.

Lyndell King

Clarity in the Midst of Chaos

My morning was off to a bad start at the convalescent center where I worked as a registered nurse. The night nurse was not feeling well and had left early; she hadn't finished her work. Two nurse aides didn't show up, so we were even more understaffed than usual. That left me with a team of two nurse aides unhappy with their overloaded assignments and a licensed practical nurse. We had fifty-seven residents on our unit, most of them completely dependent. I expected a new admission at any time.

We each took a hallway and began getting patients out of bed and prepared for breakfast. We changed wet beds, washed and dressed residents, and helped them into wheelchairs. Once we got everyone to the dining room, most of the residents needed someone to feed them. To say it was hectic would be a mild understatement. The administrator paced up and down the corridor, heaving loud sighs. He didn't offer to help. If he intended to imply he saw a bunch of incompetents running around, no one had time to be offended. The staff, such as we were, would readily admit we looked like panicky rodents scurrying around in a maze.

I glanced at my watch. I was already over an hour late dispensing the morning medications. Every available staff person had gone to the dining room to help residents with breakfast. My stomach clutched with anxiety. I hadn't even begun the real work of the nursing profession—treatments, medications, and calls to doctors. I hustled down the hallway toward my medication cart. From the corner of my eye, I caught a glimpse of Lawrence Galowich. Larry had numerous ailments: congestive heart failure, severe arthritis, and senile dementia, to name a few. He could take a few unsteady steps with a walker, but he preferred his meals in his room. Apparently he had been overlooked in our frenzied rush, and no one had served his breakfast tray. I made a mental note to check on that. Larry's burly frame filled the doorway of his room. Bushy white eyebrows hovered over his gray eyes. "Hi," he said, grinning pleasantly. That typified Larry, confused but always cheerful.

I stopped short and took another look at the scene. Larry wore only the top part of his blue pajamas, nothing else. The rest of his body was completely naked. The disposable protective underpants he should have been wearing lay crumpled and unused by his bed. Larry had not made it to the bathroom. A professional observation wasn't required to recognize that he desperately needed a shower, immediately.

"Oh, no," I grumbled. "Not now."

I wondered why I had to be the one to find him. Larry couldn't help his incontinence, but his mishap was definitely ill timed. Actually, I would be hard-pressed to think of a good time. I had no choice but to hold everything and give Larry a shower.

I spotted a woman from the housekeeping department in the hallway. I gave a frantic call to her and asked for some help.

"It isn't my job to clean up the messy stuff," she sniffed. "Housekeeping only sanitizes the floor."

I was unaware we had such a defined division of duties, I thought facetiously. I wanted to yell, "Hey, I could use some help here." Instead, I grabbed some paper towels and proceeded to wipe the smelly substance off the floor the best I could. Once that was done, I motioned for the housekeeping woman to take care of "sanitizing" the disaster area. Now, I had only Larry to contend with. He stood grinning like a happy child delighted to receive my attention. I threw a bed sheet over a wheelchair, plopped Larry in it, and covered him with the corners of the sheet.

With the speed of a marathon runner, I rolled him down the hall to the shower room.

Larry is a big man, so it took all my strength to lug him from the wheelchair and plunk him onto a shower chair. I tossed his pajama top into a hamper and turned on the water full blast. The force of the water made the long shower hose dance around like a silly snake doing the rumba. Water sprayed in every direction, flooding my shoes and saturating the pant legs of my white uniform. Larry giggled. Damp but undeterred, I managed to scoot Larry near the running water, grab the hose nozzle, and spray him. While I soaped, scrubbed, and shampooed him, Larry hummed.

Once he was squeaky clean, I struggled awkwardly to get him into a sweat suit. His stiff body was cumbersome and unyielding. After what seemed like an endless tussle of pulling and tugging, I finally had him dressed and back in the wheelchair. Aware that the morning was already wrecked and that I'd never catch up, I gave him a quick shave and combed his hair.

"Larry, you look terrific," I said when I finished.

Larry did look good. His nurse was another matter. The small shower room was hot and humid. My hair hung limply around my face, and my glasses were smeared. Laundry hampers filled with reeking linens surrounded me. Sweaty and grubby, I certainly didn't smell like fragrant lilacs. Both my deodorant and my stamina had been severely tested.

Larry treated me with one of his generous smiles. "You like what you're doing," he declared.

It was the first rational statement I'd ever heard from the eighty-seven-year-old man, whose chart indicated progressive dementia and Alzheimer's disease. I looked into his face. Larry's eyes reflected innocence and gentleness. His startling words reminded me of why I became a nurse. I wanted to have meaningful contact with people, and I wanted to make a difference in some small way. Suddenly my chaotic morning became worth every effort.

"Yes," I responded. "You're right. I love my job." I leaned down and gave Larry an affectionate squeeze on his shoulder. "It is going to be a good day after all. Thanks, Larry."

Barbara Brady, R.N.

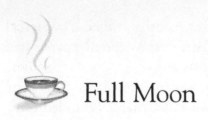 Full Moon

I was in a patient's room monitoring the ventilator when I felt my pager go off in my pocket for what seemed like the billionth time that shift. Some nights I felt like a walking switchboard, and already, only a few short hours into the shift, it looked like it was going to be one of those nights. I was relieved that I had switched the pager to vibrate, so it hadn't disturbed the patient, who was finally sleeping peacefully after receiving a shot of morphine. I stepped out of the room and checked the number on my phone; the page was from my favorite nurse.

"Another C-section," Karen said when I called her. "And all the delivery rooms are full too."

"Must have been the hurricane," I said. Though all the nursery nurses were attributing the busy night we were having to the full moon, I thought it had more to do with the tropical storm that had swept through our area nine months earlier. Power had been out for three days, and I figured people had resorted to other recreation.

"If we keep up this pace, we're going to run out of luck," I said to Karen. We had already attended three deliveries together, and we had another seven hours to go in the shift. "Odds are, we're going to have a hard delivery or a sick baby before the night is over."

"This one is just a routine failure to progress," she reassured me. "We should be in and out of there in no time."

"Sure hope so. I've got three open hearts to wean from respirators and two ventilator patients in the cardiac unit," I said.

"Meet you back there," she said.

When I got to the OR suite, I quickly scrubbed and gowned, and began to prepare the infant-warming room adjacent to the operating room. I peeked through the window and saw Karen gowned and waiting to catch the baby. I quickly checked the ambu bag and suction equipment, and then cranked up the heat to ninety. Newborns like it tropical.

I peered again through the window while I sent up my usual prayer, that this new life would have a healthy start. The smell of cauterized flesh always kept me from entering the OR unless I absolutely had to. It was difficult enough for me to watch a belly sliced from ten feet away. I made eye contact with Karen every few minutes. They say the eyes are the windows to the soul. This time, with Karen, they were doors flung wide open to a delivery nurse's worst nightmare. The cutting finished, the doctor reached in and pulled out the baby. I didn't hear a cry.

No cry. That was my cue to rush to my side of the warmer. Karen hurried over and placed the newborn down on the warmer. While I dried and stimulated the baby, Karen grabbed the cord and felt for a heartbeat.

"No heartbeat," she said.

I grabbed the ambu bag and started forcing air into the baby's lungs, praying this was just shell shock and not something else. Something I couldn't and didn't want to imagine. While I gave the baby oxygen, Karen listened with her stethoscope for a heartbeat.

"Rising," she said.

I kept forcing air in.

"One hundred," she said.

But the baby was motionless. Still no spontaneous respirations.

"Did the mom get drugs?" the neonatologist asked as he brushed past me.

I had been so focused on doing my job that I hadn't noticed the extra nurses or the anesthesiologist enter the room. Within minutes, the neonatologist placed a tube into the baby's throat to facilitate easier breathing. While I continued to bag oxygen and air into the endotracheal tube, we transported the baby to the special care nursery, where I hooked her up to a ventilator.

The mother was taken to recovery; the dad was led to the neonatal intensive care unit. He stood helplessly next to the bedside looking at his new daughter, unable to hold her in his arms. He touched her hand ever so gently with his finger and watched as another neonatal nurse searched the infant's tiny arm for a vein to insert an intravenous line.

"What's her name?" Karen asked.

"Nevaeh," the dad said.

"How should I spell that?" she asked.

"It's 'Heaven' spelled backward," he said. "She's our gift from Heaven. Our angel."

I wanted to hug him, to tell him God never sends more than you can handle, but I'd learned and been told that it was best to keep my faith to myself at work.

My beeper went off again. I was being called to the cardiac unit to adjust the settings on the ventilator of a middle-aged woman who had suffered a massive heart attack. I made the changes the doctor ordered and checked on my other adult patients. My pager went off again.

"Room twenty-four," Karen said and hung up.

I ran. A call for assistance in a room delivery can be anything: a stuck baby, a bad strip on the monitor, or a mom in trouble. Plus, you never know how many people will be in the room. Room deliveries were not my favorite.

I stood at the side of the warmer and again sent up a silent prayer.

"Nevaeh's mom just came in to see her," Karen whispered. "It was awful. She sobbed so hard."

I nodded. The one saving grace of my job was that, unlike my patients and their loved ones, once the crisis is over, I walked away. I never allowed myself to think it was walking from one tragedy to another.

I heard the doctor instruct the mom to push, and then I heard a cry. A screaming baby boy was placed on the warmer. Karen smiled at me.

"Come here and meet your son," she told the new dad.

He beamed as Karen placed the father's new little bundle from Heaven into his arms. "You have the best job in the world," he said.

Again, I felt my pager go off and left the room.

Five hours later at shift change, I gave report to the coworker taking over my patients, and the shift supervisor.

"Nevaeh is the baby on the vent," I said.

"What kind of a name is that?" the shift supervisor asked.

"'Nevaeh' is 'Heaven' spelled backward," I explained. "The baby's dad said she is their gift from Heaven, their angel."

"So? 'God' spelled backward is 'dog,'" he snickered. "Who names their kid that?"

Ignoring his comment, I continued with the report.

As I walked to my car, I remembered the father's troubled, yet thankful, face as he touched his newborn daughter's tiny hand. I took comfort in knowing that, despite his worry, his faith would sustain him through the arduous hours and days ahead. Then another father's face, filled with joy as he held his newborn son, appeared in my mind. A smile crossed my lips and my eyes brimmed with tears as I remembered his words: "You have the best job in the world." I looked up at the sky, at the full moon setting in the west as the morning sun rose in the east, and something deep inside told me all would be well with Nevaeh.

In the dawn of that new day, I also realized that my work didn't consist merely of dealing with tragedy after tragedy. It was also about witnessing miracle after miracle.

Linda Lee Hanson, R.T.

The Importance of Being Harold

onnie hummed as she made her first rounds of the evening shift. So far, everything was going smoothly, and she took that as a welcome sign that tonight was going to be less hectic than last night.

"Oh, no!" Connie gasped as she entered Harold's room, the sight of him jolting her memory.

Harold Regan was a big man, more than six feet tall and built like a locomotive, and he had a personality to match. Friendly and outgoing, he was like a fresh breath of spring, and all the staff had taken a liking to him.

Harold had been admitted to the hospital for observation and tests following an episode of chest pain and shortness of breath at his workplace. For the first few days of his hospitalization, he had worn a portable heart monitor while he underwent the tests and walked around the hospital unit pursuing the normal activities of daily living. The monitor had been removed the previous day, leaving a sticky residue where the leads had been glued to his chest, back, and limbs.

"Do you have anything that will get this tape and gunk off my skin?" Harold had asked Connie when she checked in on him during her first rounds. "It's sticking to my pajamas and everything."

"Sure," she had told him. "I'll bring some remover back on my next round."

But then there had been an emergency at the far end of the unit that had tied up much of the nursing staff for more than an hour. Followed by a frantic rush to catch up on the rounds of administering medications and completing treatments while the nursing assistants handled the routine care. Followed by mounds of paper work. And it was past midnight by the time Connie had dragged her weary body out of the hospital and headed for home.

Now, as she looked at Harold smiling at her, the memory of his simple request flashed back to her, and shame flushed her cheeks.

"I'm so sorry, Mr. Regan, for not getting back to you last night. We had this emergency down the hall, and . . . well, I'm really sorry.

"Did someone remove the adhesive for you today?" she asked hopefully.

"No," Harold answered. "Everyone was too busy. But I took a shower and put on a clean shirt, so it's not quite as sticky now."

"I truly am sorry," she repeated.

"Oh, it's okay. It wasn't that important."

"But it was important to you," Connie said. "I'll take care of it right now. I'll be back in a flash."

She practically ran to the supply closet. She grabbed a bottle of adhesive remover, a handful of gauze squares, and a clean pajama top, and rushed back to Harold's room.

During his brief hospital stay, Harold had been friendly and talkative, constantly chatting with and teasing the staff as they went about their duties. Now, he was uncharacteristically stoic. As Connie gently rubbed and scrubbed to remove the rubbery residue clinging to the skin on his chest, back, and upper arms, he sat silently in the chair, staring straight ahead at the ball game on the television. When she asked whether she was being too rough, he responded with a barely audible "no ma'am." After a few unsuccessful attempts at conversation, Connie left him to his ball game and worked silently, but the change in Harold's demeanor distressed her—and she blamed herself.

His feelings are clearly hurt, and who can blame him? she thought. *I'd be upset, too, if my nurse had forgotten all about me.*

When all the goo was finally removed, Connie gently wiped away the adhesive remover with a warm, wet washcloth and then patted his skin dry with a clean towel.

"That ought to do it," she said, handing Harold the clean pajama top. "And again, I'm really sorry about yesterday."

As he stood and slipped on the shirt, he turned to Connie and said softly, "This is the first time in my life that anyone has acknowledged that something was important to me."

Suddenly, he reached out with his massive arms and folded her against his barrel chest in a bear hug that nearly squeezed the breath out of her. Just as suddenly, he released her, but not before she noticed the dampness rimming his eyes. Speechless, Connie watched as he dropped into the chair and turned his attention back to the ball game. She swiped at her own tears as she gathered her supplies and slipped from the room.

When Connie made her last rounds, she was happy to find that Harold was back to his jovial self and looking forward to being discharged the next day. She, however, was changed forever. In the years that followed, whenever a patient had a seemingly trivial request, Connie thought of Harold and was instantly reminded of how a little thing can make a big difference in a patient's care.

Marilyn J. Hathaway

Cloudy with a Chance of Sunshine

Startled by the sudden outburst of music, I groped for the snooze button until at last there was silence. As I lay there resisting the urge to roll over, I reviewed the list of patients I was scheduled to see. I'd start out with Mr. Murphy, who needed his insulin injection. Then I'd make my way over to the Cables. Hopefully, the new medication would have kept Mrs. Cable's pain under control. I wasn't sure which was worse, watching Mrs. Cable stoically put up with her discomfort or sensing her daughter's helplessness in being unable to prevent her mother's pain. With any luck, there would be enough time before lunch to do the initial assessment on my newest clients, George and Sadie Knoff, an elderly couple who lived on the edge of town.

Slipping into my housecoat, I went to the bedroom window and opened the curtains. The sky was gray and dreary. The street below was already humming with activity. A woman wearing a pin-striped suit and heels scurried into a BMW. *What would it be like to trade places with her for a day of corporate glamour?* A hint of envy tugged at my conscience as I stumbled into the bathroom to shower.

With little time to spare, I grabbed some fruit for the drive and ransacked the closet until I finally emerged with an oversized umbrella. Stopping at the doorway, I examined my appearance in the mirror. For a fleeting moment, I caught sight of a poised graduate nurse donned in a starched white uniform and cap. I looked more closely. The memories of human suffering staining my expression drew a sharp contrast to the crisp white dress. I shook my head to clear the disturbing image and left for work.

At 10:45, pleased with how smoothly my morning visits had gone so far, I pulled over to the side of the road to review the referral sheet for my next appointment: *seventy-eight-year-old woman with Alzheimer's being cared for by her husband. Assess level of coping.*

Since it was my first visit with the couple, I decided to call to let them know I was on the way. The phone rang at least a dozen times before I hung up; I rechecked the number and dialed again. Finally, a man answered, clearing his throat several times before saying hello in a raspy voice. I introduced myself as the community nurse that was scheduled to meet with him and his wife at eleven o'clock. A lengthy pause followed. Finally, Mr. Knoff murmured that it wasn't really a good time for visitors, but he hesitantly agreed to meet with me. I couldn't help but wonder how welcome my visit would be.

I pulled into the driveway of the small bungalow a few minutes later. The grass on the front lawn grew sparsely and was marred with heavy patches of dandelions ready to disperse more seeds at the first hint of a breeze. A tangle of branches from a large, overgrown shrub protruded onto the front walkway. I rang the doorbell and waited while a thin, scruffy tabby cat, eager for attention, rubbed its neck on my leg. Finally, Mr. Knoff, appearing hurried, answered the door and quickly shuffled me down a dimly lit hallway and into the living room. He promptly asked if I would excuse him while he finished assisting his wife.

I sat down on the couch and scanned the room. The telltale clues of George and Sadie's secret existence began to emerge. A thick plastic sheet draped the seat of the armchair by the window. A cloudy glass of water with the settled remnants of a pill or two stood on the adjacent end table. Outdated newspapers were scattered across the coffee table, held in place by the crusted remains of a TV dinner.

I got up and approached the fireplace. A lovely picture of George and Sadie embracing graced an arrangement of family photographs. At the end of the dust-covered mantel was a card that caught my eye. Yellow with age, it appeared well worn, like a favorite novel that has been read over and over again. The inscription inside read,

> *George: You have blessed my life with so much.*
> *All I have to offer you is my undying love. Sadie*

"I'm very sorry to keep you waiting." George's voice could be heard coming down the hall. "We're running a bit late this morning. Had a difficult night; I must have slept in."

George came around the corner, gingerly ushering his wife into the room. Thin and fragile, bearing little resemblance to the woman in the photograph, she clung firmly to her husband's arm.

"That's quite all right. You left me in good company," I said, glancing down at the cat, who was still vying for attention. I turned to Sadie, extended my hand to her, and introduced myself. Making no attempt to take my hand, she eyed me suspiciously.

"Have you come to put me away?" she asked, the tone of her voice defiant.

With a flushed face, George patted his wife's arm. "Now, now, Sadie, you worry too much. We don't need to worry about that, do we?" His voice faltered slightly as he spoke.

"No, Mrs. Knoff, I haven't come to put you away. I came to see if we can provide some services that will help your husband care for you, here, in your home."

George led Sadie to the plastic-coated armchair by the window. "That's good, that's good. That's good, isn't it, George?" I watched quietly as George reassured and fussed over her, making her comfortable.

Completing the history and physical examination proved challenging. Sadie's memory was obscure, and she often seemed detached from the conversation. Eventually, she drifted off to sleep, but not before George had tucked a pillow at the side of her head. I was grateful for the opportunity to speak to George alone.

"Tell me what it's like for you, George."

He paused a moment and then glanced back at his wife before speaking. "She's my life. I have to do this for her." He swallowed hard. "You know, I spent forty-five years driving a bus, and when I dreamt of retiring, I never pictured anything like this."

George went on to describe his life, how he lived in fear that she would leave the stove on or wander outside at night. He admitted to knowing very little about his wife's disease. What he did know was that her condition had deteriorated significantly over the last year. She now needed help with even the most basic things—bathing, dressing, eating, and toileting.

"Do you have any family or friends to help out?"

"Our son lives out of town and can't afford to visit often. As for friends, well, it's difficult for them. The visits get further and further apart, until they stop coming around at all. I used to love the company."

"When was the last time you were able to get out on your own?"

"On my own?" George rubbed his forehead. "Not for at least the last six months. I used to be able to leave Sadie at home and run an errand or two, but not anymore."

I sat for a moment admiring the courage and strength of the man before me. I could appreciate the weight of his responsibility. It was the same weight that left me feeling heavily laden on most days. The difference was that he couldn't lay down his burden when his shift ended; his shift was twenty-four hours a day, seven days a week, 365 days a year.

"George, what keeps you going?" I had to know.

He sighed softly. "Well, it's all in how you see things. Like when the weatherman reports it will be cloudy with a chance of sunshine, you can either assume it's going to rain or hope for some sunshine. Every day that Sadie knows who I am is like a ray of sunshine."

Blinking to clear the tears, I took a few much-needed moments to gather myself together. I pretended to rummage through my bag for the correct form until I felt able to speak. Then we discussed the opportunities for assistance. Together, we formulated a plan that would provide Sadie with the personal care she required as well as help for George with managing the meals, shopping, and housework. As I stood to leave, George stood, too.

"Thank you, for everything," he said, extending his hand to shake mine. "I had no idea this type of help was available. Just being able to talk with someone, I feel like a weight has been lifted."

I clasped both his hands in mine.

"I think we both gained something from our visit, George. One thing I've learned is that I won't be needing this today," I said, waving the umbrella in the air.

Yes, it's all in how you see things.

Dorothy Wright, R.N.

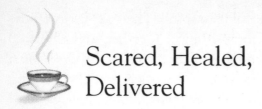

Scared, Healed, Delivered

Three and a half years had passed since I lay in the same metal bed, gripping the same rails, staring at the same ceiling, waiting for a baby to be born.

My first labor and delivery experience had been well planned. Seven days after my due date, the family doctor had scheduled labor to be induced. As I walked with my husband past the nurses' station to an assigned room, it was as if I were the only woman in the hospital coming to have a baby that day. The halls were so quiet I could almost hear the snow falling softly outside.

Fifteen hours later and long past the calm feeling I had had coming to the hospital, my sweat-covered arms held a newborn boy.

I would see several nurses during my forty-eight-hour stay. The older, grandmotherly nurse who told me to lean toward her as the epidural needle stung my lower back; later, she would hand me my son, swaddled in a blue-and-white hospital blanket. The young rookie nurse who confessed she was scared of long needles and would never have pain medication with her labor. The cheerleader nurse who snatched up my son and showed me how to get a good burp out of him; she also insisted I get up on my feet and walk the halls despite my postdelivery discomforts. All of these nurses came to visit me during the low points, when I couldn't get the baby positioned correctly at the breast or when I felt like passing out after going to the bathroom. My sleep-deprived, pain-med-induced stupor kept me from remembering these blessed nurses' names.

Then a petite woman wearing glasses walked into my room.

"I have a few things to share with you before you leave," she said with an Irish lilt.

The woman was my discharging nurse and had been assigned to instruct me on everything from changing a dirty diaper to preventing breast engorgement once I got home.

"My name is Monica." She held a spiral-bound notebook about the size of a cookbook. She proceeded to go through this parenting instructional manual, section by section, answering even the most complex baby-related questions with a soothing you-will-do-fine type of voice.

I was already dressed to leave the hospital and had only to change my son into his coming-home outfit. A hospital stay that had started with such predictability, right down to the amount of Pitocin I'd needed to start contractions, was ending with an enormous amount of confusion, as I wondered how the hospital staff could now expect me to take care of a baby. Without their help. Still, with her gentle voice and simple explanations to my most outlandish questions, Monica was a source of calm that comes from being a nurse with true empathy.

After settling our son into his car seat and packing our things into the car, my husband and I waved good-bye to this nurse who had guided and reassured us.

More than three years later when I arrived back at the same delivery ward, the circumstances couldn't have been more different. My labor started at home on a warm summer morning, and by evening, my husband was hurriedly wheeling me down the hall to the nurses' station.

I couldn't understand much of the conversation that my husband had with two nurses about my age. It turns out that my first pregnancy and birth had pre-cipitated a progressive hearing loss that made some speech difficult to understand. As the two nurses met me in the delivery room, their steady voices and direct eye contact made it apparent that my husband had told them I was hard of hearing. When epidural time came, one of the nurses used hand gestures to show how I should lie when the needle was inserted.

After my daughter was born, I was taken to a recovery room and greeted by a different attending nurse every few hours. They all seemed to mumble, though I tried to listen to their words closely. Finally, I broke down.

"Please speak up," I politely asked, "because I have hearing loss, and the hospital noises are too loud for me to understand you."

They cautiously nodded their heads and gave me a brief look that questioned why a thirty-year-old can't hear well. Then they re-explained themselves a little louder. Already tired from the round-the-clock feedings with my daughter, I was also exhausted from the combination of labor and having to lip read whatever every new nurse who came into the room said.

By the last day of my hospital stay, I had had it with trying to compete with the sound of loud hospital air conditioners as I listened attentively to soft-spoken nurses ask me questions I couldn't hear.

"Hello. I am Monica."

The nurse with the Irish lilt and nurturing smile made her way to my bedside. The same calm voice.

"How are you feeling?" Her voice was no louder than a whisper, and her accent was as defined as before. So, one would assume I wouldn't be able to understand her and would have to repeat the hearing-loss speech again. Amazingly, not only could I hear every word she said, but I could also respond with assurance.

"I'm fine," I answered.

Her familiarity was eating at me.

"I remember you," I said. "You were my nurse when my son was born three years ago."

"Oh." She smiled. "That was a long time ago."

I filled her in on the details of my expanding family and how proud my husband and I were to now have a son and a daughter. I told her about the hearing loss, although I assured her I could hear her with no problem.

"I never would have known you couldn't hear well," she said with warm eyes.

That afternoon, holding my new baby daughter in my arms, another nurse wheeled us to the elevator and out of the hospital. I showed my son his new baby sister as he waited with Daddy in the hallway. As the elevator descended to the ground floor, I thought about Monica, the woman with the lilting accent, friendly eyes, and reassuring words—the nurse who helped me to believe, twice, that everything would be fine.

Shanna Bartlett Groves

A Measure of Worth

As I read the brief, but telling, history of yet another suicidal young patient on the psychiatric unit where I work, my heart ached. I felt tears welling up in my eyes as I wrote out the assignment sheet. It wasn't only the suicide attempt that bothered me, though that was horrific enough. It was also what had led to the young girl's desire to take her life: abuse and neglect. As a psychiatric nurse, I saw it day after day after day . . . same story, different faces . . . kids who had been beaten, raped, and traumatized in ways that could destroy a grown adult, much less a vulnerable child. Constant exposure to such human wreckage didn't lessen its impact on my spirit, though. My shift had just begun, and already my heart was sore. Sometimes I wondered whether I was doing these kids any good at all. Sometimes I wondered whether my job was worth all the heartache and turmoil.

As I handed out small white paper cups of pills to the patients, I spotted the new girl from the corner of my eye. I could see the angry purple slash on her neck where the scarf had been. She hung back, head down, eyes averted. I saved her meds for last and walked over to her.

"I'm Miss Donna," I said softly. "Let's sit down and talk while you take your medicine."

As the girl and I sat across from one another and she took her medication, I struggled to think of something to say that might break the ice, to let her know I was there to help her, that she could trust me. Suddenly a memory flashed before me—of me, sitting in a hospital much like the one where I was now a nurse. I was thin, dying thin, and didn't want to eat; I was also depressed, making for a potentially lethal cocktail: one shot of depression, two shots of anorexia, coming up. I remembered feeling incredibly lost and displaced. Just that morning my roommate had tried to stab me in the chest because the "voices" had told her to, and then I had gotten caught stuffing quarters in the pockets of my robe to fake weight gain. I felt like I was in the wrong place, in a dungeon locked in with "real" crazies, when all that was wrong with me was that I needed to cheer up and put on a few pounds.

Then Chad, one of the nurses on the ward, had walked over to me. Chad reminded me of Katharine Hepburn—she had bright, intelligent eyes, a mane of tousled red-gold curls, rosy cheeks, a wide-open grin, and a no-nonsense manner. She sat beside me and touched my hand gently.

"Donna," she said gently, "could you please take your medicine, and then we can talk for a while?"

For the rest of my hospital stay, Chad was my hero. She treated me like a person, not just a patient. She was direct in her approach, like Kate Hepburn, but always considerate and respectful. I talked with her every chance I got. When I was down, she was there, and we talked through all the underlying issues that my anorexia and depression were helping me to mask. I considered her my mentor. I wanted to be like her: strong, caring, and confident.

It had been years since I'd thought of that time, so long ago it sometimes didn't seem real. I looked at my young patient and recognized the hopelessness, distrust, and fear in her eyes. I knew that the slump in her shoulders and her icy silence were walls she had put up to keep from getting hurt again. I decided to tell her my story, no holds barred. I told her about Chad, how her belief in me had helped me to believe in myself, make healthier choices, and turn my life around.

In sharing my experience with this troubled girl, I realized something else, something I didn't share with her, because she was still too fragile to hear it. I realized that I might not have made it had it not been for that wonderful nurse who took the time and made the effort to reach out to me personally. And that is when I realized what I'd been doing wrong in my job: I'd neglected to see my patients as people, each with their own histories, needs, and desires. Instead, I had pooled them all together into one endless sea of misery.

I reached out and touched my patient's hand. This time when I spoke with her, I really looked at her. I didn't see just another "oppositional defiant disorder slash ADHD" case; I saw a frightened young girl with a broken heart. I couldn't undo or erase the horrible things that had happened to her. But I could be there for her now. I could listen and help her to heal. I could show her I cared and believed in her. I could help her to believe that she was beautiful, important, and loved. I could make a difference, a real difference, in this girl's life, and maybe, just maybe, that difference would change or even save her life.

Making a difference. That is why I got into nursing in the first place. It is why, no matter how tired I get or how many times I have to duck into the bathroom to cry, I will keep on being a nurse. It is worth it, because my patients are worth it. That is what I learned many years ago from a wonderful nurse named Chad, who thought I was worth saving and healing. Now I get to return the favor.

Donna Surgenor Reames, R.N.

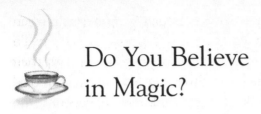

Do You Believe in Magic?

Several years ago I tried to retire from my almost forty-year nursing career. After living in Chapel Hill, North Carolina, for seventeen years, my husband and I decided we needed a break from the muggy weather and headed west to a small, artsy town in Wyoming—7,000 feet up the flanks of the magnificent Wind River Range. We'd spent count-less weekends camping and hiking at Hanging Rock State Park, north of Winston-Salem, North Carolina, and looked forward to hiking the seemingly endless terrain that surrounded our new home of Dubois.

This lifelong flatlander thought she had landed in paradise. Getting up at the crack of dawn, we'd drive to any one of the thousands of trailheads and hike all day, stopping for a picnic lunch and photo shoots of the purple mountain's majesty, a lone new-born fawn, or a field of wild iris. We'd climb up to peaks so lofty it felt as though we were walking on the top of the world.

The closest hospital was eighty miles away, so it looked as though my retirement was safe. Then, I met Meghann. Walking down the street one morning and minding my own business, I passed a girl in a wheelchair. She had what looked to be, and was, a feeding tube taped to the side of her face. As I exchanged good mornings with her mother, Meghann smiled. By the end of the next week, I'd become a residential habilitation trainer to the twelve-year-old ex-preemie with spastic quadriplegic cerebral palsy and severe mental disability. I tried to convince myself that I wasn't exactly a nurse.

Meghann and I became fast friends. We listened to 1950s rock-and-roll while baking chocolate chip cookies, played Barbies, and watched Michelle Kwan, Scott Hamilton, and Elvis Stojko figure skate on TV. Though Meghann's body and mind were greatly impaired, her pure spirit was very much alive and lovely beyond angelic.

I'd worked in pediatric and newborn intensive care since the 1970s and was embarrassed by the morbidity of so many of the preemies we'd sent home. Preemies like Meghann.

A month before I met her, Meghann had barely survived a planned two-hour orthopedic procedure that turned into a fourteen-hour fiasco. When all was said and done, Meghann couldn't swallow. She tried to go to Heaven twice during the surgery and then again a day later, but it wasn't her time to leave us. Perhaps because there was something she wanted to do first—swim with the dolphins.

Meghann's doctor informed the Make-A-Wish Foundation about Meghann's wish, and her ordeal, and they decided to make her wish come true. Meghann and her guests would get to swim at Dolphins Plus, a therapeutic dolphin-encounter program in Key Largo, Florida. In addition to her mother, Meghann could choose a friend to accompany her. She chose me.

When we arrived at the lagoon, a therapist fitted Meghann with a life vest and gently positioned her in the cool water while her mother and I sat on the deck and watched. The pod of dolphins swam by and then circled the therapist who was holding on to the young teenager with spastic legs and arms. Meghann's cerebral palsy usually causes people to look away; the dolphins had no such inhibitions and studied her. Circling her again, the pod swam closer. One lingered much closer than the others, murmuring in beeps and bleeps.

"His name is Charlie," said the therapist, "and he's nosey."

Meghann followed him with her eyes. The clicks of his sonar seemed to penetrate her heart. Now just inches from her face, he peered into her eyes. Meghann blinked, but continued to watch her new friend. The dolphin turned slightly and brushed his body against her spastic legs.

"Yeah!" Meghann shouted in excitement.

Charlie circled again. Then he drew closer, gently pressed the length of his body against hers—and something happened. Something magical. Meghann's legs relaxed, and the grimace of a grin she normally wore when happy gave way to a soft, pretty smile. It seemed as though Meghann's brain waves were resonating with Charlie's.

Suddenly he dove deep, turned quickly at the lagoon's bottom, and soared upward. Up, up out of the water he shot until his whole body was exposed in an arch. As he slipped back into the water, he splashed her with a tap of his fluke.

Meghann jerked and her eyes opened wide with surprise, as the salt water dripped from her face and hair.

"Charlie only splashes people he likes," the therapist explained.

Meghann relaxed for a moment only to tense up again as the pod returned and encircled her. Charlie had called the others to Meghann's side, and now seven full-grown dolphins hovered around her.

"A personal introduction," said the therapist.

One by one, the dolphins filed by Meghann, bombarding her with their sonar vibrations, freeing her spastic muscles and filling her soul with a sense of both security and euphoria. Meghann squealed with joy and clapped her hands, oblivious to all that surrounded her—except the dolphins.

Charlie moved forward from the pod. He pushed his nose against her foot, then against her knee, and then against her hip.

"Yeah!" Meghann yelled again. "Yeah, yeah, yeah!"

Meghann swam with the dolphins once a day for three days. I swam with her on two of those sessions. On the third day I opted to stand ashore and take photographs. Watching the healing magic between Meghann and the dolphins, I thought about my career and wondered whether I had ever been able to do what the dolphins had done. I hoped I had.

On the last day, the dolphins swam by in single file, close enough for Meghann to reach out and touch them with the arm that usually couldn't be straightened. Charlie lingered at her side as though he was her protector—or her best friend. The fragile girl swam in that soothing environment with seven huge mammals—and she was not afraid. Her face glowed with peace and happiness. She didn't seem to notice that for those fleeting moments she was no longer spastic; all that mattered was the communion of their souls.

Charlie, the inquisitive dolphin, had done what few humans dare to do. He investigated Meghann from head to toe. He gave her unconditional acceptance. He introduced her to his friends. He saw her pain and responded to it with healing love. Was Charlie a better nurse than me? I wondered.

The music of the dolphins, their high-pitched whistles and squeaks and clicks and beeps, are etched forever in Meghann's memory. At the mere mention of the word "dolphin," her whole being lights up with gladness and she shouts, "Yeah!"

I've always tried to be a caring nurse, but sometimes even the most promising treatments result in compromised lives. The dolphins helped me accept that the best I can do is give unconditional, loving care in the hope that it will transcend the constraints of this world and cause all my patients to say "Yeah!"

Shelia Bolt Rudesill, R.N.

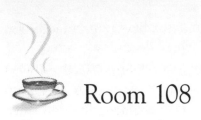

Room 108

I didn't know. Not when my parents were dying and in hospice care. Not when I later became a hospice volunteer and visited dozens of clients in both homes and nursing facilities. I didn't know what it might feel like to be a patient in a hospice bed until I experienced it myself.

Her touch feels warm as she holds my hand gently between hers. I turn my head on the pillow and meet the eyes of Sandy, the patient care manager. Her compassionate face focuses on mine and wordlessly conveys her empathy. A wave of intense emotion rises within me, and I avert my gaze to the floor.

Although Sandy is seated, her head is higher than mine, as are most of the objects in the room, which somehow makes me feel smaller. Looking up from my horizontal position on the bed reminds me of how vulnerable I am, lying here in room 108 of a hospice house, a place where death is expected.

My senses are heightened, and everything around me is vivid. Sandy's image is framed by the glass patio doors behind her. The deep purple of her dress matches my mood. Backlit, she appears outlined with a golden aura. It seems appropriate that she should look so angelic. Outside the sun shines on a crisp autumn day. While leaves are turning color and dropping, roses still bloom in the landscape, a mix of life and death, indoors as well as out.

The texture of the blanket brushes against my cheek. I am covered from toes to chin, and it feels as though I am shrinking into a cocoon of bedding. *Is that what death will be like, a metamorphosis of a sleeping larva in a cocoon? Will I emerge into the next existence like a butterfly with the sun glinting off iridescent wings, free to dance on the wind?*

Ten years ago I held my dying mother's hand as she lay in a bed much like this. That was my first contact with hospice care. Only fifteen months later I felt my father's hand grow cold in mine. I wonder what thoughts they had as they looked up at me from pillows, waiting for death to release them from disease.

Only once do I recall my mother asking, "Why did this happen to me?"

Filled with anticipatory grief, I told her, "We will all die from something. You got breast cancer. What I do know is that every time you go for radiation or chemotherapy treatment, you have a joke to share with the nurses and technicians. They chose a career helping people, many of whom will not survive their illness. That must be very difficult. But Mom, you always arrive with a smile on your face, brightening their day and reminding them why they do their job." I told her that the staff—buoyed by her pleasant, upbeat attitude—would then transfer that positive energy to their next patient. And that patient, in turn, would go home and perhaps smile a bit more and make life easier for caregivers and family.

"You are like ripples on a pond," I said to her. "You have no idea how many lives you are affecting because you have cancer. Long after your death, you will still be touching lives."

Tears filled my mother's tired hazel-brown eyes as she whispered, "I like that."

Months after her death, I walked my father down the hall of the same medical building for his first chemotherapy, feeling a weight heavier than anything I'd ever experienced in my life. I couldn't go in with him that time, as tears overwhelmed me.

One of the nurses who remembered my mother joined me in the hallway. While hugging me, she explained to another patient's family member, "Her mother was one of our favorite patients. She was always so cheerful. We still have a cartoon she drew for us on our bulletin board."

I looked where the nurse pointed, and sure enough, a pencil drawing with my mother's signature was posted in a place of honor. I smiled softly and thought, *Ripples on the pond, Mom. You're still touching lives.* How could I have known those months before that she would be touching mine on that dark day.

Though I longed to repay my debt of gratitude for all the hospice organization had done for my family, it was several years before I found the courage to become a volunteer. The training program rekindled a spark in my wounded spirit.

I selected my first family visit assignment based solely on the coincidence of the patient's first name being the same as my mother's. While the patient's daughter and I got acquainted, I discovered that the young woman had worked as a nurse's aid in the facility where my mother had stayed. She remembered taking care of my mother and seeing my father and me there. Now, our roles were reversed. I couldn't imagine a clearer affirmation that I was following the path I was intended to take.

People have often asked me, "How can you stand to do something so depressing?"

I tell them that each time I accept an assignment as a family visitor, I know I'm about to embark on an incredible journey. Someone approaching the end of life needs some support or service I can provide, and all it involves on my part is some of my time and a lot of my heart. My time with a patient and his or her family might be spent holding hands and listening to life stories. Sharing roses from my yard with a gardener confined to bed. Reading Scripture to someone whose vision has faded. Being an appreciative audience to a patient playing favorite tunes on a harmonica. The simple act of offering a sip of water or half a teaspoon of food for someone who has become too weak to manage it alone. Tears will be shed, of course, but we will also share laughter—and life.

Yes, creating a special bond with someone who is terminally ill and watching that person suffer and decline, and then saying goodbye, is hard. And there are moments when I fret that what I do is not enough, and moments when I struggle for the right things to say to my patients and their loved ones. But I always feel enriched and honored by these experiences.

As I lie on the hospice bed in room 108, I am engulfed by the memories of all those patients, and I wonder whether they knew how much I treasure the gifts they bestowed upon me. They were teachers, even in their final hours, and their legacy is marked not by the deterioration of their bodies but by their positive influence on other people. I wonder what legacy I will leave behind. *Will the world be a better place because I lived in it? Will I leave ripples on the pond?*

I glance back up at Sandy, whose caring gaze has never wavered. *Does she know what I am thinking and experiencing right now?* She certainly has sat at the bedside of many hospice patients. But I doubt that anyone who has not been in that bed can truly know what it is like.

A voice from behind me breaks the spell.

"I think we've got what we need," the photographer says. "You can get up now."

Sandy smiles and releases my hand. I toss back the bedding and sit upright in the bed. The director of public relations for the hospice house stands in the doorway, nodding approval. The photographs will be used in a brochure being created for the grand opening of the new Alexander Cohen Hospice House.

I swing my feet out of the hospital bed and walk out of the room. Only a few minutes had passed, but it felt like a lifetime. I hesitated and looked back over my shoulder at room 108, realizing that I had just learned one more lesson from my hospice patients.

It's not always about knowing the right words to say. The silence of those moments, as I lay still in the bed with Sandy holding my hand, allowed me the opportunity to examine deep feelings. Human touch made me feel anchored safely as my thoughts drifted to emotional memories. I will now be more comfortable with the silence of my clients and their families, as I quiet myself and become their anchor.

Roberta McReynolds

Divine Intervention

I remember Liz Hood well. She was the nicest nurse in the ward where my mum was recovering from surgery.

On my daily visits with my mother, I could plainly see that the hospital was short-staffed. Most of the nurses were working extra shifts, and I knew they must be tired. It also seemed to me that some of the patients were quite difficult. The hospital had no air conditioning, and the weather was extremely hot and muggy that July, which no doubt made everyone a little irritable. One patient in particular, a girl of about thirteen, seemed especially cross and petulant.

On the morning of her admittance, the young girl criticized and complained virtually nonstop, demanding this and that until the nurses grew weary of trying to placate her and all but ignored her. When she rang for a nurse yet again, Liz Hood went over and sat on the edge of the girl's bed. She calmly asked what the problem was and then listened patiently to a litany of complaints.

"Is this your first time in hospital?" Liz asked when the girl had run out of gripes.

"No, and the one I was in before was wonderful compared to this, and so were the nurses!" came the response.

Liz nodded, validating the child's opinion. Then she said, "So, I suppose you don't want to be a nurse then."

"Are you crazy? Of course not!"

"My father thought I was crazy when I first told him I wanted to be a nurse . . . and he was very angry," Liz began her story. "He had already arranged for me to attend commercial college to become a secretary; he had spoken to my high school teachers and my mother but not to me. My father was not the sort who took kindly to a defiant child, but I knew so strongly in my heart that nursing was what I wanted to do that for once I was not afraid of him.

"So, I enrolled myself in nursing school, forging his signature on papers. I used to climb out my bedroom window and go off to extra classes. It was a few months before the commercial college contacted him and asked why I had never attended any of the classes."

Interested now, the young girl stared at Liz. "So what happened?" she asked. "Did he get mad?"

"Mad, oh, he got mad all right. My dad had an awful temper."

"You must have been pretty upset," the girl offered.

"Yes, I was. I felt hurt and distressed to realize that my father looked down on something that was so important to me. I tried to explain that I thought it was noble to look after those in need, but he never understood. He felt nursing was a profession for people of lesser station in life, and he prohibited me from returning to nursing school."

"How did you do it, then?" the girl asked.

"Well, I did a year at commercial college, and then my father had a serious heart attack. When he came out of hospital he was so full of praise for the nurses who had looked after him that he relented. Personally, I think it was divine intervention; I had been praying relentlessly for God to help me follow my dream to become a nurse. Now, here I am!"

"But is it still your dream? I mean, you all run around emptying bedpans, serving food, cleaning up yucky stuff, dealing with grumpy people . . . like me," she said sheepishly, smiling for the first time.

"Is it still my dream? Yes, it is. Is it just as I'd dreamed it would be? Not always. Sometimes, like today, when we're short-staffed and it's hot and everyone is on edge, and I'm exhausted from working extra shifts and trying to appease unhappy patients, it can be difficult. But I still love being a nurse."

"Anyhow," Liz said, as she patted the girl's hand and then stood up. "What was it you wanted?"

"Oh, just something to drink; I can't reach my juice."

"No problem," Liz said, promptly pouring the juice into a glass and handing it to her young patient.

I was impressed by the way Liz had handled the situation and was eager to see whether it would stop the girl from being so demanding. When I arrived the next day, I was surprised to find the young girl's bed empty and asked my mum if she had been discharged already.

"No, the poor soul passed away last night. Something went wrong, and they were all flying around but were unable to save her."

"How awful," I said, staring over at the empty bed in disbelief.

As I watched the nurses scurrying to make up the bed and prepare for a new patient, it occurred to me that perhaps they were too busy to be upset at her loss. Then Liz Hood came along and walked over to the empty bed. She stood silently for a moment, her head slightly bent as though she were sad, and then she touched the bottle of juice still standing on the bedside table.

Mum told me later that when the girl's parents had come to pick up her things, the father had asked for Liz. He told Liz that his daughter had talked glowingly about her, saying she was the best nurse she'd ever had. He thanked Liz for taking the time to tell his daughter her story and for making her last day a bit brighter than it might have been.

A few weeks later, after having watched Liz Hood comfort so many different patients, I casually said to my mum's nurse, "I can't understand why that nurse hasn't been promoted to a higher position."

The nurse glanced over at Liz and smiled. "You wouldn't want to know the offers she has turned down. She could be the senior nurse on staff by now, but she always turns them down."

"But why? She is so good at what she does."

"Exactly," the nurse agreed. "She is good at understanding patients' fears and worries. She's good at talking with them and helping them deal with difficult situations. She's an excellent nurse, and she is absolutely content with that. Don't you think she is one of the luckiest people alive?"

"Oh, yes," I said. "Lucky, indeed."

That Liz Hood has been able to do work she was meant to do, that she enjoys doing and does so well, is certainly her, and her patients', good fortune. Or perhaps it is, as this exceptional nurse claimed, a matter of divine intervention.

Joyce Stark

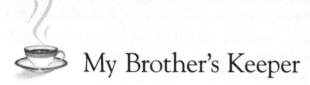

My Brother's Keeper

"Nurse, Nurse, Raoul's having a seizure. Come quick."

Jumping to my feet, I maneuvered around wheelchairs and walkers, sidestepping slow-moving campers, until I reached the front of the room. Sure enough, Raoul was in the throes of a generalized onset tonic-clonic seizure right in the middle of the makeshift stage. Men with developmental delays and physical disabilities gamely stepped around Raoul as they continued acting out the lines they'd rehearsed for their Valentine's Day skit. Just another Friday afternoon at Camp Costanoan, they seemed to say. In their special-needs world, seizures were more common than rain showers, and the show must go on.

Six feet four and weighing more than 200 pounds, twenty-two-year-old Raoul was a formidable sight as his muscles flexed and extended in response to the wild electrical surges in his brain. Turned to his side with his head cushioned among a pile of jackets that had been quickly donated by fellow campers, Raoul was well protected. Juan, his equally massive brother, crouched watchfully at Raoul's side and raised a hand in greeting when I arrived.

"It's the same thing he does at home, Nurse," Juan said.

Raoul's color was good, and his seizure was following its usual pattern, so I knelt on the floor beside Juan and watched as the convulsions softened and then tapered off. As Raoul's muscles relaxed and his breathing deepened into a snore, camp staff helped me roll him onto a gym mat and pull him to the side of the stage. Juan followed along, patting his brother's back with awkward grace and murmuring reassuringly whenever Raoul opened his eyes.

Later that night, I made my way to the brothers' sleeping cabin for one last check before bedtime. Lying on adjoining beds with their dark hair glistening from their showers, Raoul and Juan looked up at me with expressive dark eyes.

"Thank you for taking care of my little brother, Nurse," Juan articulated slowly but precisely.

With a lump in my throat, I told Juan what a wonderful brother he had been to Raoul during the seizure.

"I try to be, Nurse," Juan responded with heartfelt humility.

Throughout the next day, a Saturday, I frequently caught sight of Raoul and Juan engaged in the camp activities. They painstakingly glued colorful hearts onto lacy cards to take back home to their mother. They awkwardly played basketball with fellow campers on the sports court, and patiently reenacted a particularly difficult charade for the guys in their lodge. At mealtimes, the two brothers sat side by side, carefully passing the serving platters back and forth with their large hands.

Each time I handed Juan or Raoul his tiny plastic cup of anticonvulsant medications, both of them would reply, "Thank you for taking care of us, Nurse. Will you be at the dance tonight?"

My answer was always the same: "Wouldn't miss it for the world."

As darkness fell I slipped into the main lodge where the dance was already in full swing. Each camper had a unique style and a peculiar grace: A tall young woman with autism bounced up and down in solitary enjoyment in the center of the dance floor. A man with microcephaly and severe mental retardation rocked quietly back and forth beside his counselor. An older man in a wheelchair grinned as his counselor pushed and pulled the chair in time to the rock beat. A group of women with Down syndrome twirled while their eyes sent a silent invitation to several men with developmental delays.

In the far corner of the room, Raoul and Juan stood awkwardly, their hands straight at their sides like soldiers, facing Margaret, an attractive redhead with mild developmental delays. Well groomed and socially competent, she was clearly the catch of the evening. Both of the brothers were smitten with Margaret, bewitched by her bright red lipstick and flowing dress. Margaret, who lived at home with her elderly parents, was clearly enjoying her evening as the belle of the ball. Her eyes sparkled as she first touched Raoul lightly on the arm and then peered up coyly at Juan through lowered lashes. With their freshly shaven cheeks and handsome profiles, Raoul and Juan were ready to party. But what to do about this dilemma: two brothers and only one of the beguiling Margaret? Glancing at one another uncertainly, Raoul and Juan were clearly at a loss.

As the rock tune ended and the strains of Simon and Garfunkel's "Bridge over Troubled Water" filled the room, Juan abruptly gestured to his brother and pulled him away from Margaret. Expecting an altercation, I watched as Juan murmured quietly to Raoul while touching his brother gently on the cheek. Then, Juan tipped an imaginary hat in Margaret's direction before turning to choose a partner from the group of women with Down syndrome, and tears filled my eyes. Raoul strutted back to Margaret and gallantly held out his forearm to lead her onto the dance floor. As Juan and his chosen partner shuffled slowly past the spot where I was standing, he smiled and pointed to Raoul.

"My little brother is dancing, Nurse."

So many times, nursing takes place within the four walls of an institution, in brightly lit rooms filled with complicated machinery. But camp nurses know that medications are only a small part of life, that treatments can be delivered in the pool or on horseback, and that emergencies occur in the midst of skits. Camp nurses provide the background expertise that allows individuals with special needs to enjoy life to its fullest.

Sandy Keefe, R.N.

This story was first published as "I Am My Brother's Keeper" in *Nursing Spectrum/Nurse Wire*, February 2004.

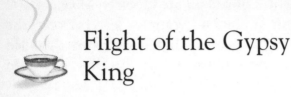

Flight of the Gypsy King

When I worked in Boston in the 1980s, there lived there a substantial population of Eastern Europeans called Romani, whom locals commonly referred to as "travelers" or "Gypsies." At the time, I was amazed to learn that this fabled group actually existed. When a Roma became ill and all traditional folk remedies failed, this insular group put aside their fears of contamination by non-Gypsies in order to seek modern medical treatment, somehow intuiting how to navigate the complicated health-care system.

One day an elderly Roma with a large family was admitted to the general medical unit at a renowned teaching hospital, where I was a staff nurse on that unit. In his early seventies, the patient, who was suffering from advanced cancer, had recently become bedridden and weak. His family had cared for him for as long as they could, but he had reached the point at which nothing more could be done, in their world or ours, to treat him. His breathing was labored and at times shallow, and he was fading in and out of consciousness. His family had brought him to the hospital to die, knowing we could take measures to make his passing more comfortable that were unavailable to them.

Not surprisingly, family members stayed by his bedside. What was unusual was that he was surrounded not only by his immediate and extended family, but also by the other members of his clan—round the clock. He was obviously the patriarch of this Roma clan.

I'd heard about Boston's Romani population before; an 800-bed facility is fertile ground for such urban tales. It was rumored that Gypsies wandered around the hospital looking for equipment and wheeled out the small metal carts loaded with TVs and portable cardiac monitors, boldly passing right by security guards, too shocked to catch them, in broad daylight. So, with dozens of Gypsies wandering the floor at all hours, distrust was palpable. Female staff carefully locked up their purses. Even the med students hung on to their stethoscopes. Everyone was slightly on edge.

Some of the Roma group spoke heavily accented or no English; many of the older members relied on the young for translations. Most were solidly built, including the women, and all had dark eyes and thick, lustrous hair. A few could have used a good bath. Some of the women were well dressed in long, flowing skirts, scarves, and shawls, while others of the group wore the mismatched, ragged outfits of street people.

We nurses had little physical care to perform for our shared patient, as he was washed and comforted by a constant rotation of female clan members. It was difficult to establish a rapport with the group, as the faces kept changing. At times, there were up to fifteen people in the room. They would just appear, babies and children in tow, even after hours, and we wouldn't notice until they were spilling out into the hall. We arranged with the clan's spokespersons that their visitors could congregate at the nearby visitor lounge and that six at a time could stay in the room.

As any nurse knows, a marked turn for the worse rarely happens on the day shift, while eager residents are available to respond to crises. I was charge nurse on the evening shift when the Gypsy patriarch's condition worsened, with failing heart rate and loss of responsiveness. I alerted my supervisor, who arrived to check out the situation at the same time that several burly Romas began rolling our moribund patient's bed, with him in it, down the hall toward the elevator.

"He is our king. He must die under the stars," said one of the men, appearing anxious and agitated.

My supervisor managed to stall them while I called security. This was against all hospital policies and regulations. We couldn't allow a dying patient to leave our floor like that. *Take him outside? While he was in the process of dying? When it was they who had brought him to the hospital to die in the first place?* How absurd that seemed to us.

Our translators returned from the lounge, we explained why we could not allow a dying patient to just be wheeled outside, and thankfully the standoff was quickly diffused. Our oblivious patient was returned to his room, and we sat down to talk with the group's spokespersons, who then explained their dilemma.

The eldest daughter of the gypsy king explained that they knew death was near. They were a nomadic people; they disliked and mistrusted the confinement of closed buildings. In their belief system, it was necessary for him to die under the open sky so that his spirit could be released. It was also essential for all the relatives, who had continued to arrive from across New England, to be near him upon death or at the very least to be able to visit his bedside. Honoring this tradition was important, not only as a duty to their dying elder, but culturally and spiritually for the group.

A compromise was struck: Visitors could continue to visit the Gypsy king through the night in groups, and he would stay in the room if we could open the window. That way, his spirit would be able to slip out of his body peacefully and not become trapped in this world.

Our unit, which was located in a new tower section of the hospital, had a state-of-the-art air-filtration system. Because of the sophisticated ventilation system and because the unit was on the ninth floor, all windows were sealed shut. My nursing supervisor swung into patient advocate mode, calling a laundry list of engineering and maintenance supervisors. She was insistent: at least one window in the room must be opened immediately.

Meanwhile, the numbers of the king's visitors continued to increase and to rotate through the area. So far, the group had been peaceful and cooperative, and we wanted to keep it that way.

How are they slipping through security at this hour? I wondered. It occurred to me that perhaps they did have a secret route into and out of the building, bypassing the main entrance. I've since read that among their many qualities, Gypsies are proud of their ability to adapt to any environment. They certainly seemed resourceful that evening, with their uncanny ability to appear and disappear.

Eight hours flew by, and still our Gypsy king held on to life—and still the window remained closed. As I tended my other patients and escorted the Romani visitors into and out of their leader's room, my supervisor doggedly climbed the authorization ladder until she finally got permission for the seemingly simple request: an open window.

That's when the smoke alarm went off. Candles had been lit in his room by a well-meaning visitor. Other patients were curious about the hubbub; I explained the situation as best I could and closed as many patient doors as possible. Idle med students and staff from other parts of the hospital strolled through; the whole place was abuzz with the news: the king of the Gypsies was dying. Our normally quiet floor had become a circus.

The head of maintenance appeared, looking baffled and hassled, toolbox in hand. With a few well-placed whacks of hammer and chisel, the window frame was released and the smoke alarm deactivated. Soon, the Gypsy king quietly passed away by candlelight, his head next to the open window, his spirit able to escape from his body and rise to the stars and beyond.

I went home late that night, tired but satisfied. It is said that hearing and awareness are the last senses to leave our bodies when we die. The Gypsy king waited until we were able to grant the conditions he desired for his death. Even when someone's beliefs may be hard for us to fathom, human understanding and cooperation can transcend our differences. We're all just people, after all.

Mary Ellen Porrata, R.N., A.P.R.N.

A Beacon in the Storm

For several years I was employed at a veteran's hospital in middle Tennessee. As the nurse coordinator, I wore both a clinical and a managerial hat, with administrative responsibility for the psychiatric ambulatory care clinics and clinical responsibility for a large caseload of clients that I was seeing in psychotherapy. Most of my clients were Vietnam veterans who suffered from post-traumatic stress disorder (PTSD). I worked closely with these veterans as well as with their families, who also were impacted by their loved one's illness.

The facility where I worked made a concerted effort to educate surrounding communities about services that were available from the Department of Veterans Affairs. One venue used for this purpose was community health fairs, where I would talk to veterans and hand out literature about our programs.

The main subject I focused on was PTSD, its symptoms and available treatments. Even though the Vietnam conflict had ended more than two decades earlier, many veterans had never sought treatment for PTSD. This was not surprising, given that two of the primary symptoms of PTSD are fear of being around people and distrust of any government institution. My objective in attending the health fairs was to establish rapport with vets who perhaps needed assistance but were reluctant to come in on their own and to convince them that we had help to offer them.

One such fair was held at a Veterans of Foreign Wars hall in a small town in middle Tennessee. It was a success in that we had approximately 300 attendees and there were long lines at my table most of the day. We had opened the doors at 8:00 in the morning and were scheduled to close at 4:00 that afternoon. By 3:45, I had given out most of the educational material I'd brought and the number of people coming to my table had slowed down.

I leaned back in my chair and looked around the room. I noticed a man looking at me rather intently. I had seen him sitting in the waiting area across from my table earlier but thought nothing of it. His facial expression now was tense, and I could tell he was uncomfortable. I smiled and nodded hello to him. He hesitated for a minute and then got up from his chair and walked over to my table. I invited him to sit down and introduced myself. I asked if he was a Vietnam veteran and whether he had ever received treatment from the VA before. He acknowledged that he was in Vietnam during the Tet Offensive in 1967, but said that he had never sought any treatment . . . until now.

I asked him to tell me about his life and what had happened to him since Vietnam. He spoke of being raised in a mountain community in eastern Tennessee by parents who'd had to scrape to make ends meet. He was the oldest of six children, and had been drafted into the Army at age eighteen. After a year in Vietnam, he received an honorable discharge from the military and returned to his childhood community.

Life after Vietnam had not been easy. At first, he got a job working for the sanitation department in his hometown but had difficulty relating to coworkers. He had recurring nightmares and difficulty sleeping. In an effort to get relief and rest, he started drinking. When he realized that was causing problems, he stopped using alcohol as a crutch, but the nightmares continued.

He'd married a girl he had known in high school, and that was not working out well. He admitted it was his fault, because he had trouble with trust and intimacy. His wife, though, didn't understand him, and so blamed herself for the problems in the relationship. They were still married, but he spent most of his time staying in a one-room cabin he had built in the woods.

Other relationships in his life had also continued to deteriorate, and eventually he lost his job with the city. Unable to hold a regular job, he eked out some money by finding and selling arrowheads. His life was becoming increasingly unraveled, and he had seriously considered suicide. He told me he didn't see much hope for his future.

I asked him what had made him decide to seek help now, after all that time. He asked if I remembered a certain veteran who had been in one of my groups, and I told him I did. He said the man, who was a friend of his from high school, had encouraged him to come to us and said that we could help him. I told him we would do our best. I scheduled him for a physical exam with a doctor at the medical center and an appointment with me for the following Wednesday at 2:00. He promised to be there. I hoped he would be.

On Wednesday, 2:00 came and went, and he was nowhere in sight. I worried that he had scared himself out of coming. Then, at 2:30, I saw him through my office window walking hurriedly toward the clinic building. I was there to greet him in the waiting room as he rushed in, short of breath and apologizing for being late. He explained that they hadn't quite finished with the physical, but he told them he had to "go see that lady because he'd promised he would."

During our counseling session, we talked in greater detail about his nightmares and difficulty sleeping. I suggested a few basic relaxation techniques, recognizing that he had a long way to go to heal his wounded soul. But it was a start, and he said that taking this first step and knowing he could talk to someone about his difficulties made him feel a little better. He confided that he'd struggled over whether to talk with me at the health fair. He said he had arrived at 11:00, but couldn't work up the nerve to come over to my table and had almost left several times. By the end of the day, he'd decided to just leave without talking to me.

"What made you change your mind?" I asked.

"You smiled at me."

During my forty years as a nurse, it has been experiences such as this that have taught me not to take the seemingly small things for granted, both in my professional and personal life. We never know when a smile, a touch, a reassuring hug, or an attentive ear will be the beacon that lights the way to safe harbor.

Linda Swann Dumat, R.N.

On the Other Side
of the Bed

After fourteen years of working in the critical care division of a large university teaching hospital, I thought I had seen it all. I had been through two nursing shortages and one cutback. In fact, the "cushy" job I had finally managed to earn, working Monday through Friday, 7:00 A.M. to 3:00 P.M., as a hyperbaric nurse, was eliminated. Suddenly, I found myself back in bedside nursing. Signs of burnout started to show. I came, did my job, and went home; I didn't try to make a difference in anyone's life. I was looking forward to an Easter vacation with my kids in Florida.

A few days before my much-needed spring break was to begin, as I was leaving a tanning salon, I was met at the door by a policeman. He informed me that my twelve-year-old son, J.J., had been badly burned. My mind reeled: *How could that be? He was home with his dad and sister.* The officer could tell me only that my son had been burned severely after pouring gasoline on the charcoals of our barbecue.

Later I would learn that my husband had started the charcoals to grill hamburgers, and then he and my daughter had run out to rent a movie, leaving my son, who had stayed home sick from school that day, at home. While his dad and sister were gone, J.J. went outside to check on the coals, and thinking they had gone out, he grabbed the gallon gasoline container used to fill the lawnmower and poured it on the hot coals. The gas fumes ignited and flames shot back toward the container. Instinctively, J.J. dropped the tank, and it exploded between his legs.

I raced home and found the paramedics loading my son into the ambulance. I climbed right in after him; the ambulance driver told me to get in front, but I just ignored him. When I got into the back of the ambulance with J.J., he looked at me and said he was sorry. He told me he had remembered to "stop, drop, and roll."

"Am I burned badly?" J.J. asked. "My legs don't hurt."

One look at his legs and I knew why they didn't hurt: the burns were third-degree, full thickness. I slipped immediately from mom to nurse mode, taking control. Having worked in a burn center for ten years, I was able to assess the situation. I quickly calculated the size of the burns and the IV rate.

When we arrived at the hospital's burn unit, nurses with whom I had worked several years earlier ushered me in and treated me like old times. I slipped on a pair of scrubs, a mask, and gloves and followed my son to the admitting area. The burn doctor came in and asked me to leave.

"No. I'm staying," I barked.

"Okay," he said, frowning. "But just sit there."

The burn doctor examined J.J. and assessed the size of the burn; his calculations matched mine. I was amazed that I could still figure burn size without the need of a chart. The burns were photographed by the medical photo staff. The nurses took J.J. to the tub room to debride the burn, and then washed and dressed the burned area. For two hours, my son endured this painful and frightening experience, while all I could do was hold his hand and reassure him he would be okay.

After we finally got J.J. tucked into his hospital bed, the severity of the situation hit me. He had a full-thickness, third-degree burn over 35 percent of his body. Though my son was receiving the proper care and his odds were good, the only thing I could think of were the patients I had taken care of who had been horribly disfigured or disabled by their burns, and a few who had not survived them. That's when I slipped back into mom mode and realized what side of the bed I was really on. I wouldn't be going home after my shift. My shift had just become twenty-four hours a day, seven days a week, and it would last for four months.

Suddenly, I had to rely on others to make the right decisions, to anticipate problems, and to care about what was happening to my son. I was scared at first, but at the same time, I knew these doctors and nurses were the best in what they do. I put trust, and my son, in their capable hands.

He was hospitalized for the first month, and during those four horrific weeks, I saw the "art" of nursing in a way I'd never seen it before. Every morning the nurses would give J.J. his pain medication before his bath and take him to the tub room to wash the burns, remove any of the dead tissue, and redress the wound. He began to dread waking up in the morning. He could never eat his breakfast, knowing what was coming. After his bath, the physical therapist would come and work with him for about an hour. All of this was very painful, and after the morning ritual he would sleep for half the day.

Colleagues to whom I had once taught burn care now taught me that patient care goes beyond nursing techniques and procedures. It also means including and thinking about the patient's family. They would allow me to help with J.J.'s care at night, when they reinforced his dressing before he went to sleep. They brought in a cot so I could sleep in the room with him, and they encouraged me to leave for short times when J.J. needed his privacy or I needed a break. Of course, I didn't want to leave his side at all, but they assured me they would call me and let me know how he was doing. Once, my husband stayed with him while I went home overnight. True to promise, one of the nurses called me to let me know J.J. was fine.

"I'll take care of him as though he were my own child," I'd heard more than one member of the staff say.

And they did. They even sat and played video games with him the times when I went to work for a few hours. They brought him candy and new video games. They were also there for me, giving me a sounding board when I needed to express my anger, frustration, and fears, sorrow, and happiness. They showed they cared about me as a mother and a person.

My son recovered very well from his burns. He returned to school, where he was active in sports, and he played all four years on his college football team. Now twenty-three, he sometimes goes to the burn unit to counsel young children who have been burned.

When my son was finally well enough for me to go back to work, I returned to the bedside recharged and with a more positive attitude. I have always been a strong patient advocate, but after my son's hospitalization, I became a strong family advocate as well. I always include the patient's family or significant other in any treatment plans or problems. Now, I'm the one who promises to take care of the son, daughter, mother, father, or other loved one as if he or she were my family. I can see the same relief in their eyes that I felt when those words were spoken to me.

Constance R. Shelsky, R.N., C.C.R.N.

R$_x$ for the Best Worst Christmas

rowing up with a father who was a police officer and a mother who was a nurse, I considered working on holidays a fact of life. Even though we frequently had to celebrate our holidays before or after the actual day, I never heard my parents complain. They passed down a philosophy that if you choose to enter a profession of service to others, you can expect to make some personal sacrifices.

While my brain accepted this concept, my heart still sank when the December schedule was posted and I saw that I was scheduled to work the 11:00 P.M. to 7:00 A.M. shift on my first Christmas Eve as a registered nurse. I was accustomed to attending midnight mass with my family, and for the first time, I would be the one who missed out on a family tradition because of my work schedule.

As is the case at most hospitals, December brought an onslaught of delicious treats from physicians, patients, and families. As the holiday drew near, the census on the GYN unit to which I was assigned dwindled. Very few women scheduled surgeries of a nonemergency nature so close to Christmas. There was even talk of closing the unit entirely, if all of the patients were well enough to be discharged on the twenty-fourth, thereby eliminating the need for me to work. With my fingers crossed, I called to check in with my supervisor on Christmas Eve. I was informed that only one patient remained on the unit, but since she was still receiving IV antibiotics, she would be spending the holiday in the hospital. Her physician had refused the hospital's request to temporarily move his patient to another area, so I was going to be doing private duty.

I have to admit that my attitude was less than festive as I counted down the hours until I needed to leave for work. Feeling much like the Grinch with a heart two sizes too small, I clocked in shortly before eleven and got report on my solitary patient. The 3:00 to 11:00 P.M. nurse was out the door in a flash, anxious to get home to her waiting family.

With flashlight in hand, I made my way down the dark and silent hallway to check on my lone patient. The room was darkened, with the exception of the lights twinkling on a small artificial Christmas tree on the nightstand. Expecting to hear the sound of quiet breathing, I was surprised to hear a soft sniffle. Putting on my best nurse face, I asked whether something was wrong.

My question opened the floodgates, and she poured out her heart to me. It seemed that I wasn't the only one experiencing the disappointment of spending Christmas Eve in the hospital. I pulled up a chair and turned on the lights. She looked at me with a tear-streaked face and apologized for my having to work that night. After a few minutes of commiseration, I decided to take the bull by the horns. Here we were, two young women spending the holiday together by a twist of fate. Where was it written that I had to spend my night at the nurse's station while she spent the night alone in her room?

I dashed back to the kitchenette and returned with the remains of that evening's party. After pushing the two beds closer together, I set up a make-shift buffet of goodies on an over-bed table and found a radio station playing Christmas carols. We spent the night nibbling on our feast and sharing stories of Christmases past. The local television stations helped out by running Christmas movies throughout the night. During commercials I performed my nursing duties, taking vitals signs and hanging piggybacks.

As morning approached, my charge began to yawn. I cleaned up the evidence of our holiday party and turned off the television. As she settled down for her long winter's nap, I returned to the nurses' station to complete my charting. The house supervisor stopped by to see whether I had survived my boring night, and I assured her all was well.

Shortly before seven, I checked in on my new friend one last time. She sleepily thanked me for making her Christmas Eve special and keeping her company throughout the long night. As I slowly made my way back up the long hallway I realized that, indeed, Christmas had arrived. And just like in Whoville, it had "come without ribbons, it had come without tags, it had come without packages, boxes, or bags."

Over the years I have worked many holidays. Never again have I experienced the sense of true caring that I experienced that first Christmas when my heart grew three sizes overnight.

Mary E. Stassi, R.N.

Lessons from 3-West

When I graduated from nursing school, I applied to work days in the psychiatric ward of St. Patrick Hospital. I was hired for night shift on 3-West, the medical floor. To say it was an adjustment working nights and sleeping days was an understatement. The transition from the cushioned, supervised world of student nursing to "team leading"—supervising other caregivers and patients—was overwhelming.

As I struggled through those stressful, sleep-deprived days, I kept hearing the voice of my instructor, Marie Bradley, echoing in my mind.

"Everyone should start out on a medical floor," she said. "You'll learn so much."

Little did she know that the lessons I'd learn on 3-West had as much, if not more, to do with living than with nursing.

Two months after I started working at St. Pat's, a day-shift position opened. Because of my limited seniority, I didn't apply. Neither did anyone else in-house. A nurse new to the hospital and our area got the job that could've been mine.

Lesson #1: You can't win if you don't try.

In October, when an evening-shift position was posted, I applied and got the job. Seniority, however, came into play during the holidays. Being the most recent hire on the 3:00 to 11:00 P.M. shift, I was scheduled to work both Christmas Eve and Christmas Day.

I lived six hours from my family; this would be my first holiday alone. I bought a small tree and decorated it with two strands of lights, shiny ornaments, and tinsel.

Returning home from work on December 24, I found a wrapped box propped between my screen and front doors. The gift lifted my melancholy mood until I noticed there was no tag. *Maybe it's at the wrong door.* I turned over the box, and the rattle from within first startled and then scared me. After turning on every light in my modest apartment, curiosity got the best of me, and I unwrapped the box. A jolly, painted wooden chef holding wooden spoons grinned at me from his resting place. Seeing his broad smile and rosy cheeks made me smile, too.

I gazed over at the gifts under my tree. Our family Christmas tradition is to open one *gift Christmas Eve and the rest Christmas Day. Open them by myself tonight or by myself in the morning?*

Tonight.

I opened all my gifts and put on my new nightgown and pearl ring. They made me feel closer to my family.

Christmas morning dawned to below-zero temperatures. When I tried to start my car to go to Mass, the gas in the tank was frozen. I blinked back tears and prayed the gas would thaw before I had to drive to work that afternoon. A phone call from home later that morning lifted my spirits. By the time I had to leave for work, the gas in my tank had thawed. I drove to work thinking that at least I'd be able to share dinner in the cafeteria with other hospital employees—such that there were. The parking lot was nearly vacant, and I discovered why when I got to 3-West: We had only thirteen patients. Thirteen patients meant we needed only one R.N.: me. Being the lone R.N., I could leave the department just long enough to grab food from the cafeteria and bring it back to the nurses' station. I dined alone in our break room.

Lesson #2: Extend an invitation to the lonely during the holidays.

In April, I moved to day shift. We changed our staffing model from "team leading" to "primary care." One morning just after the beginning of my shift, my patient, Mrs. Larson, who was recovering from an above-knee amputation, lay writhing in pain. Forty minutes after I'd medicated her, her pain was still unrelieved and she was restless when Dr. Springfield made rounds.

"Give her fifty of Demerol IM," Dr. Springfield said as we walked together to the nurses' station.

"Fifty?"

"Yes."

I hesitated. Mrs. Larson was a slight eighty-year-old woman. Fifty milligrams of Demerol on top of the narcotic I'd already given her seemed too much for her petite stature.

"Now," the doctor ordered.

My stomach knotted as I removed the Demerol from the locked box. As I injected the medication into Mrs. Larson's wasted muscle, I vowed to check her frequently.

A short time later, Ursula, a fellow nurse, interrupted the dressing change I was doing in room 310.

"We need you in 320 immediately!" Her voice had an urgency I'd never heard before.

I hurried down the hall, uttering a silent prayer: "Please be okay."

Sister Henrietta stood beside Mrs. Larson's bed. "Her respirations are slowing."

I ran to the nurses' station and dialed the doctor's office.

"It's an emergency," I said to the receptionist, praying I wouldn't hear "Code Blue" announced over the intercom. "Mrs. Larson is barely breathing," I said the moment I heard Dr. Springfield's voice.

"Give her Narcan IM, one milligram—stat."

Mrs. Larson rallied after the injection. As Sister Henrietta and I watched her color improve and her respirations return to normal, my heart pounded in thanksgiving for Sister Henrietta's timely presence as I kicked myself for giving Mrs. Larson all that Demerol against my better judgment.

Lesson #3: Listen to your inner voice.

In June, Mr. Kelly, a "no code," lay dying in 302-A. Sweat beaded his brow, his every breath a struggle. His wife and daughter flanked his bed, weary after their all-night vigil.

I had bonded with the Kelly family during the two previous days and had learned that Mr. and Mrs. Kelly lived in a retirement complex across the street from the hospital. Their daughter, an R.N. from Billings, Montana, had been summoned three days earlier.

Wanting to give his family some respite and to make Mr. Kelly more comfortable in his final hours, I asked, "Do you want to go home for half an hour? I'd like to give him a bath and change his bed."

Mrs. Kelly looked apprehensively at her daughter. "Just for a bit, Mom, while Karen cleans him up."

Mrs. Kelly said nothing. She gazed lovingly into her husband's face for a few seconds, and then she leaned over and kissed his cheek. "Okay." Her voice was soft.

I squeezed each of their hands as they left the room and then hurried to get fresh linens. Back in 302, I realized that in my haste I'd forgotten a washcloth. Scurrying back down the hall, I cursed my carelessness. When I returned, it took a moment before I realized something was different. The room was quiet. A wave of nausea swept over me as I walked around the curtain and discovered Mr. Kelly's still body.

Slowly I walked toward the nurses' station. Seeing Sister Henrietta strolling toward me, the tears that had been pressing behind my eyes began to stream down my cheeks.

Sister put her arm around me and led me into an empty room. "What's wrong?" she asked.

Between sobs I choked out the words. "I—told his family—they could go—and—I wasn't even—in the room—."

Sister Henrietta enveloped me in her arms.

"And because of me—he died alone."

"Maybe he wanted it that way," she said, holding me until my sobs quieted.

Sister Henrietta stood beside me as I called Mrs. Kelly, and she accompanied me back to Mr. Kelly's room. Together we wiped his brow, straightened his sheets, and waited for his wife and daughter to return.

Lesson #4: Believe in angels on Earth. We all have our Sister Henriettas.

For twenty-six months, 3-West was my home. Now, twenty-six years later, I continue to be shaped by the lessons I learned while marching up and down that charcoal-speckled floor.

Karen Buley, R.N.

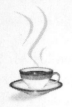

My Amazing Shift with the Handsome Dude

About ten years ago I cared for a young man in the ICU of our regional hospital. During that single, twelve-hour day shift, Shawn neither opened his eyes nor spoke a word. Yet he managed, through someone who loved him, to open my eyes.

Report revealed that Shawn was twenty-two years old. He had been born with severe physical and brain disabilities that included cranial deformities, limited intellectual abilities, rotoscoliosis, club feet, and hip dysplasia. He had never learned to walk or speak. Believing that they were unable to care for him, Shawn's parents had abandoned him at birth to family and children's services. He had become a ward of the province and lived in Sunbeam Home, where he required total care.

Shawn suffered frequent respiratory tract infections. Two days prior to being admitted to ICU, he'd been sent to the emergency room with pneumonia. He was kept in ER overnight because no ICU beds were available. The next day, with still no bed in ICU, he was transferred to the medical floor. There, he suffered a respiratory arrest as a consequence of either the pneumonia or of aspiration following some lunch he was fed.

Due to his neck deformities, both rescue breathing and intubation had been difficult. It took more than twenty minutes—too long—before the #6 ETT was successfully in place. Now, finally, in ICU, he was dependent on a mechanical ventilator, was being tube-fed, and had dopamine infusing to maintain a normal blood pressure. There were no signs that he was waking up.

Because of his legal guardianship, decisions regarding his care had to be made with the hospital's ethics committee. His code status had been deemed DNR. I was told the next decision, regarding the withdrawal of life support, would be made in a few days, following an EEG.

Shawn, stretched out on his bed, was slight but gangly at eighty-seven pounds. He was pale; his hair was dark. My first impression was that he had a sweet and peaceful face. I found huge, warm brown eyes when I lifted his eyelids to check his pupils' response to light (extremely sluggish at best). He made no response to commands or stimuli, just an odd random jerking movement of a limb. His lack of consciousness could not be explained by sedation or analgesia, because he had received neither. There were no signs of discomfort or restlessness.

His condition that day was stable at this ominous level. All he needed from me was routine care: a bath, turning, suctioning, and continuation of the mechanical ventilation, tube feeding, IV fluid, anti-biotics, and a steroid.

As I cared for Shawn, I thought about how he must have lived his days. I wondered what it was like never to have had the constancy of people who claimed him as their own, to call him "son" or "grandson" or "brother." To be at the mercy of paid and volunteer caregivers. To be harnessed into a wheelchair or to lie on a bed with his twisted spine and deformed joints. To never be able to articulate his needs or wants or to walk across a room or to make things happen. To have his body racked with coughing and to struggle with secretions he didn't have the strength or dexterity to clear himself. Surely a short life filled with so much pain had seemed long. Surely this young man had had enough. Surely it was alright if it was now over.

Our unit was hopping, and I had two other patients. I was zipping around like a pinball in a machine when a worried-looking visitor stopped me in the hall.

"May I see Shawn?" she asked.

I must have looked surprised, because this thirty-something woman felt the need to then explain that she was Kathy, Shawn's teacher, and that she'd visited previously.

I told her that of course she could see him, to go on in and sit with him. I warned her that there hadn't been much change, that he still wasn't responding but seemed comfortable.

A few minutes later, I returned to Shawn's room to do what I usually do for a visitor so obviously concerned: I put down the bedrail, made sure her chair was pulled up close so she could hold his hand, and encouraged her to talk to him, because "you never know." I shared details of his condition. Then I went about doing the "hourlies": recording the vent checks, the vital signs, tipping the urine, etc.

I remember her holding his bony hands tightly. As she watched his face, I noticed hers filled with as much love as I've seen at any bedside.

"Come on, you handsome dude; I need my hug!"

She explained to me that she always called him a "handsome dude" and that he loved it. It made him laugh.

"He has the greatest laugh in the world. Don't you, Shawn? And he loves hockey. He watches it with the other residents and really whoops it up when the Leafs or Team Canada are winning."

Kathy told me that several years before, Shawn had been a student in the special classroom she holds mornings at Sunbeam Home, but there hadn't been much he could do and his school days had lasted only three years. They had remained buddies ever since, and she sought him out every day to get one of his generous hugs.

"He also has quite the handshake," she boasted.

This was all a far different picture from the one I'd allowed myself to paint of Shawn's existence. I was ashamed at how I'd concluded his life wasn't worth living.

Kathy carried on stroking him and talking to him, letting him know how much everybody missed him. As we chatted, I learned her own children were young and in the care of a babysitter while she came from out of town to spend time with Shawn.

"He's more responsive today," she said.

"I beg your pardon?"

"He's more responsive. I think he's squeezing my hand."

I took a look. She slipped her hand back into the hollow of his.

"Squeeze my hand, Shawn."

Ever so slightly his frail fingers closed over hers.

I was dumbfounded. I told her he sure hadn't done that for me, but that a hand grasp can sometimes be only a reflex. I gave it a try with his other hand. I, too, got a very weak grasp! The rest of the world melted away. I think it was because the coals of hope had started to glow.

"Shawn, open your eyes," I said sharply.

There was a slight flutter of his eyelids.

"Open your eyes, Shawn," I repeated.

This time there was also a slight opening of his mouth. I could feel a good fight welling up inside me. I was suddenly rooting for Shawn, and I was proud of him. I wanted him to show us, to get back here and pick up where he'd left off, but healthy for a change.

If you'd walked by then, you would have seen Kathy, Shawn's teacher, on one side and Kathy, his nurse, on the other, each holding on tight to one of his hands. You would have seen our excitement. You would have known something important was going on.

What that was, as far as Shawn was concerned, I had no idea, because his EEG the next day was straight lines and his brain scan was "no flow." Life support was removed, and his breathing and heart stopped a few hours later.

I did know what was happening to me. I was learning about quality of life. I was seeing that only the person living a life can truly know the quality of that life. I was realizing that quality of life exists in the gap between expectations and reality—and the smaller the gap, the higher the quality.

Perhaps for Shawn there had been no gap. Through Kathy's few simple stories and her obviously breaking heart, I came to know a young man who, despite his difficulties, had possessed superior traits and lived a meaningful life. He had known not only contentment but also joy. He had a beautiful nature, a generous spirit, and a great capacity to give and receive affection. He'd been a loyal friend; he'd created memories. His recovery had been yearned for; his loss would be mourned. He'd been loved; he'd touched deeply. He enriched the lives of all who knew him—including, however briefly, me.

Thank you, Shawn, for teaching me. It was an honor. You handsome dude.

Kathleen Herzig, R.N.

Hubba Hubba

In July 1998, my eighty-two-year-old grandmother had to give up her apartment in the senior-citizen complex where she had lived for seventeen years. For more than a year she had failed significantly. Physical ailments came in multiples, and her memory was beginning to show signs of wear and tear, too. After many hospitalizations, our family decided that she needed to relocate to a nursing home or an assisted-living facility. My aunt and my sister researched and visited several nursing homes within a ten-mile radius. My aunt and sister—nearest to Gram in proximity—both worked full-time jobs. Gram had started requiring round-the-clock care so neither of them could have her stay at their homes.

After weeks of looking and asking many questions, word came of an opening at a fairly new facility about fifteen minutes away from her apartment at the senior complex. The Meadows, as it was called, offered a private room, congregate meals, activities, worship services, and field trips. A hairdresser would come in and do her hair. She could have all the company she wanted. The Meadows sounded ideal. It seemed like a dream come true.

Gram, however, did not share in the enthusiasm. Determined to be disagreeable, she spent much of her first two weeks at The Meadows napping. Diagnosed with depression years before, she still never understood the implications and could hardly fathom why she had no energy. She wasn't interested in trying anything that might improve her condition. She didn't want to have tea with the ladies. She didn't want to go into the parlor and hear the pianist play hymns. She made repeated comments about The Meadows being a temporary stay, when, in fact, we all knew it was to be her permanent home.

After many attempts on my aunt's behalf to get Gram to participate in one of the activities offered, she reluctantly agreed to play bingo one afternoon. My aunt knew that once Gram was in the recreation room around other people, her old sociability would return. Gram had always been a people person. Being as Gram had always been a feisty card player and lover of board games, this brought a little of her old spunk back. The real turning point, though, was when a young nursing assistant named Allen coaxed her into walking outside and sitting on the deck, and she began to accept her new surroundings.

"This is kind of pretty," Gram acknowledged while sitting on the deck.

The trees and flowers were in full bloom, and children played at the park across the street. By getting her to sample the view from outside The Meadows, Allen had struck a chord. Allen managed to get Gram out of bed on the days she said she just couldn't muster enough energy. He even helped the nurses when they dispensed her medicine; she'd always had a tough time swallowing pills.

"No, Nat," he would say, "I'll mix this in a little applesauce, and it will go down nice and easy."

Eventually my grandmother grew strong enough to go out for rides with my aunt or my sister. She always made sure to speak to Allen before she left.

"I'm leaving you, darling, but only for a little while," she'd tease as she went out the door.

"Bye, Nat. I'll miss you," he would reply, while blowing her a kiss.

She joked with the other residents at The Meadows about Allen being her boyfriend. On days when she thought he looked especially sharp, she would whistle as he walked by.

"Hubba hubba!" she would exclaim.

Allen's care for the patients at The Meadows went beyond his scheduled shift. Before he went on duty and after his shift had ended, he would visit with my grandmother and the other folks. He had a flair for fashion, and one time arranged all of Gram's outfits in coordinated sets, which made getting dressed much easier for her. Gram was very particular about how she looked.

Once when Gram was hospitalized for a blood clot in her lung, Allen went to visit her at the hospital ten miles away. He called my aunt often to inquire about Gram's condition and to ask whether there was anything he could do to help.

Gram returned to The Meadows after her hospital stay, but it wasn't long before she took ill again. Allen held her hand as they waited for the ambulance, all the while encouraging her, telling her everything would be fine. Sadly, this time Gram wasn't fine. She passed away a few days later.

Allen attended both my grandmother's wake and her funeral. We welcomed him like family. He even joined our family at my aunt's house afterward. He shared his memories of his short time spent with her and shared the tears of those whose memories spanned a lifetime.

A few days after the funeral, my aunt received a call from The Meadows. The arduous task of packing up my grandmother's belongings fell on my aunt, but she wasn't quite up to the task yet. The staff understood her reluctance.

"Take your time," they told her.

Meanwhile, Allen came to visit my aunt and offered his help, once again.

"Would it be all right if I were to pack up Nat's things and bring them to you?" he asked.

My aunt was touched by his kind offer and gratefully accepted.

Late that night, after his shift ended, Allen folded, packed, and labeled Gram's things with loving care. He organized them just the way she would have done it many years before.

Gram is missed sorely to this day. She was my confidante and mentor. She was a trusted friend to many. Yet for a long time, she had voiced her wishes: "I wish God would take me," she had said many times in her final months.

God finally answered her prayer, and in the presence of one of His servants, He answered ours as well. My peace comes with knowing in my heart that Gram was ready to go. It also comes from believing that God sent an Earth angel to help guide her along the last leg of her long, hard journey. His name was Allen. Hubba hubba, in Gram-speak.

Kimberly Ripley

Specializing Lieutenant Mulkerne

They were all heroes. That's what the young Cadet Nurses thought of the young men in their care at Cushing Hospital in Boston, Massachusetts, in 1945. The entire country had galvanized behind the war effort, but these men were among those who had fought and suffered on the front lines. These were the heroes.

The soldiers didn't act like heroes. They acted like . . . well . . . young men. They flirted and joked with the young Cadet Nurses like it was Jukebox Saturday night. On one of her first days at Cushing, a nineteen-year-old Cadet Nurse named Dot Driscoll, anxious to make a good first impression, responded promptly to a soldier who asked if she would get him a vase.

"Of course," she said. "How big is your bouquet?"

She was confused at the explosion of laughter. Another nurse explained to her that "vase" was the name the soldiers had given the urinals.

That's the way it was with those brave young men. Men who had lost limbs chided each other about not standing up when a lady entered the room. They would holler at each other to get out of bed and assist the nurses with lifting things. They joked and laughed to keep each other going. To prove they were still themselves. To distance themselves from the horrors they had witnessed. To keep the pain in their bodies and in their minds at bay. But in the quiet wards at night, when the waves of pain and the unspeakable memories came roaring back, the girls they teased by day were their lifelines by dark, their angels of mercy in white, who took their hands and guided them gently but surely back to shore.

Dot had known at the age of five that she would be a nurse. She was a tomboy with long legs, a mass of unruly blond curls, and light blue eyes. But her round little face, always ready to giggle, grew solemn whenever her family drove past the Brockton Hospital. Standing between her grandparents on the backseat of her father's Buick, Dot would point a chubby finger at the brick building.

"Gran, do you know who is in there?" she would ask.

"No, Loveen, who?"

"Poor, sick, suffering souls," Dot would chant like a southern preacher.

Gran nodded encouragingly. "Those poor, sick, suffering souls will be very glad to have you taking care of them one day."

Dot's passion became a vocation in high school, and at age sixteen, in 1940, she entered Boston City Hospital School of Nursing. Her hair was still a mass of light curls, but her knees were no longer knobby, and she received many good-natured whistles as she and her classmates walked past the Boston University fraternity houses on their way to class.

Then, after December 1941, everything changed. The country was at war, and Boston City Hospital joined the war effort. Doctors and nurses left for overseas, young men rushed to enlist, and soldiers shipped out. Dot's older brother joined the Air Force, and Dot approached her nursing studies as determined as everyone else to do her part to support her country during this troubled time. In 1942, the terrible tragedy of the Cocoanut Grove Nightclub fire killed 492 people in Boston, many of whom were servicemen on leave. Three hundred of the burn victims were brought to Boston City Hospital, and Dot and her classmates quickly learned new ways to more effectively treat victims with shock and burns.

Dot and most of her classmates joined the Cadet Nurse Corps. Dot completed basic training at Fort

Devins in Ayer, Massachusetts, where, with plenty of hard work, laughter, and some tears, all the nurses learned about military protocol and Army regulations and even mastered push-ups. At the end of basic training, Cadet Nurses were given their uniforms. Dot loved the smart gray suit with button pockets. She laid the gray velour guard's coat on her bunk and fingered the red epaulets with awe. The gray symbolized mercy, serenity, and understanding; the red strength, courage, and inspiration. The patch on the left sleeve was a symbol of the Knights of Hospitalers of Saint John, the original nurse fighting order. Dot knew she was part of something much bigger than herself. She vowed to work tirelessly to live up to the honor of that beautiful uniform, giving aid to those in need.

Dot was assigned to Cushing Hospital in Framingham, Massachusetts. The nurses and doctors, all in the Army, lived in barracks on the base. There was great camaraderie between the nurses and the soldiers in their care. Dot thrived. Her Yankee upbringing made her level-headed and practical. "Pity has no place here," she told her mother on visits home. Her Irish ancestry gave her not only an easy smile and the stamina needed for the demanding job of caring for severely injured men, but also a quick wit and sassy comebacks for the banter that characterized the wards.

The nurses treated the soldiers with respect and friendship. The soldiers, many of whom were severely injured, didn't talk about their battle experiences. That would come much later, a little at a time, confided only to a trusted loved one in a quiet voice, each humorous story triggering an achingly painful memory of a buddy lost forever. But in Cushing, it was still too close. The repartee was light and easy, and for the wounded soldiers, the nurses' companionship healed their souls even as their skillful ministrations healed their bodies. Come morning, there would be no mention of the horrors of the night. Sometimes, a look was exchanged, the soldier's silent acknowledgment of what the nurse's tender care during the rough night had meant to him, but the looks were brief and then the wisecracks started up again.

The hardest part for Dot was having her high school friends come through Cushing as patients. The first was Bobby Marshfield. Dot recognized the name on the chart but had to look again more closely to recognize the young man in the bed in front of her. The last time she had seen Bobby was at a Brockton High School football game, where he had rushed 100 yards. Now, he lay before her, older than she would have imagined, swathed in bandages, unconscious, his left leg gone below the knee.

The nurses in the Cadet Corps wore their nursing school uniforms while on duty. The Boston City nurses, in their distinctive dark blue dresses with white bibs and white hats, had the reputation for working with victims in shock and burn victims. One morning in early spring of 1945, when Dot was the charge nurse on the floor, a WAC took quick note of Dot's uniform and asked her to check on a young lieutenant in post-op. The young soldier didn't look well. Dot examined him quickly. Although many medical advances were being made at the time, pain management in 1945 was still far from being perfected. Many men died from shock, their bodies simply overwhelmed by the level of pain caused by their extensive injuries. Dot knew this was the case with the young soldier—he was in shock and had stopped breathing; his systems were shutting down. She immediately sent another nurse for the emergency surgeon and began resuscitation. The surgeon came, and agreeing with her assessment, rushed the soldier back into the operating theater to try to stop internal hemorrhaging.

Dot was just finishing her rounds that evening when the surgeon found her.

"That soldier, Lieutenant Mulkerne, made it through surgery, but that's about all I can say. He wouldn't have had a prayer if you hadn't acted so quickly. You saved his life. Now we'll see whether he'll be able to hold on to it. He's going to need a lot of prayers for that."

Dot felt elated and defiant. She had cheated death from taking one more young man. She thought for a minute of her Gran, but the surgeon's voice jerked her back.

"I'd like you to 'special' Lieutenant Mulkerne."

She went to the nurses' quarters that night feeling satisfied and strangely alone in the room full of chattering women.

For the next week, Lieutenant Mulkerne was given a private room, and Dot nursed him exclusively. His injuries were horrific. Shrapnel had damaged the entire right side of his body, starting in his back and radiating down to his hips, leg, and foot, and up to his shoulder, arm, and hand. She couldn't imagine the pain he had gone through. Dot looked at his pale face and wondered about him. He had fine features, high cheekbones, a narrow nose, and deep-set eyes. His right arm would probably be paralyzed, and the surgeon had given him short odds of ever walking again.

What had been his plans before the war? Dot wondered. *With such a face, he must be kind. He must have wanted something, a home, a family. How had he made it back this far?*

Battlefront injuries were treated at frontline hospitals. Those who survived were evacuated to England, and those who survived there were brought home. The ocean voyage from England was long and arduous for a healthy man and quite often fatal for a severely injured one. But here Lieutenant Mulkerne was, sick and suffering, but hanging on, a very determined survivor. He was twenty-three years old.

Dot chatted to her "special" lieutenant. She had a distinctive voice, her New England accent very pronounced, her voice a pleasing alto; she spoke in a low tone with a slight lilt, which emanated a calm optimism. Part of her duty was to try to bring him to consciousness, to prevent him from going into shock again and into a deep coma. She called his name, made small talk, gave him weather reports, told him silly stories, anything to keep him from slipping away again. After a week, Lieutenant Mulkerne had improved measurably, but he still had a long way to go on his recovery and was still only semiconscious when Dot's "special" rotation ended and she was transferred to another floor.

All during the week that followed, Dot's mind kept wandering back to Lieutenant Mulkerne. She wondered how he was doing. She hoped he would keep fighting. She felt like part of his fight now. He had survived so long against enormous odds, and just when his body had begun to give up, she had pulled him back.

The next Saturday morning was unusually warm for early spring in New England. The window in the nurses' cloakroom was open at the bottom, letting in cool air that smelled slightly of damp earth. Dot caught herself humming, "I'll be seeing you in apple blossom time. . . . " Walking into the ward, she saw him immediately. He was sitting up in bed, wearing a robe, still looking pale but with a trace of color in his thin cheeks. She noticed his eyes were dark blue.

"Hello" she said, going directly to his bedside. "I'll bet you don't remember who I am."

Lieutenant Mulkerne immediately recognized her voice. He looked at the pretty young nurse smiling as she stood at his bedside, and his face broke into a lopsided grin. His deep-set eyes looked straight into hers, and in a quiet but firm voice, he said, "Yes, I do. You're the girl I'm going to marry."

Cadet Nurse Doris "Dot" Driscoll and Lieutenant Donald Mulkerne were married in 1946. He received a Purple Heart and a Bronze Star for valor in combat and spent fourteen months in a veterans' hospital. He did learn to walk again. He and Dot live in upstate New York. Married happily for fifty-nine years, they have seven children and nineteen grandchildren. Two of their daughters are nurses.

Marcella M. O'Malley

A Little Love Will Do It

I stepped into the industrial-sized room with its dingy florescent lighting, sour food smells, rows of cafeteria-style tables . . . took one look at the sea of wheelchairs occupied by elderly people of varying stages of decrepitude, staring at me with watery, red-rimmed eyes, some curious, some suspicious, others blank . . . and almost turned on my heel and walked right back out.

What have I gotten myself into? I groaned inwardly.

My heart pounded wildly in my chest, and my mouth felt like sandpaper. Suddenly, my head started to spin, and my knees buckled. A strong hand grabbed my arm, steadying me.

"Are you all right?" the head nurse asked.

"I think so," I said shakily. "I don't know what happened; it felt like I was going to pass out there for a moment."

"Well, you certainly wouldn't be the first student to pass out on us," she said. "Come on, we'll go to my office where you can sit down and collect yourself."

As we walked past the throng of wheelchairs, gnarled hands reached out to touch me. I tried not to shiver. This wasn't exactly what I'd had in mind when I'd decided, at age forty, to leave a twenty-year career as a successful beautician and makeup artist to become a nurse. Now, I was wondering whether I was cut out for my new profession. There I was, a nursing student on the first day of my first practicum, and before I'd had a chance to take a single temperature, I'd almost fainted at the feet of my supervisor. The woman all the nursing students called "Bea Arthur" behind her back, because she not only looked like the actress but had the same brusque mannerisms as her TV character, Maude. The head nurse who would be judging my performance.

That was some performance all right, I thought with embarrassment. I had a feeling that my three-week dress rehearsal as a nurse in this residential nursing facility for the elderly was going to be one long, rough haul.

Fortunately, the remainder of that first day was spent filling out forms, attending workshops, and getting some behind-the-scenes instruction. By the end of the shift, the queasiness in my gut and the doubt in my mind, if not the embarrassment over my wooziness, had eased up.

The second day, each of the nursing assistants was assigned a patient for whom we would provide basic nursing care under the supervision of an R.N. I was paired up with Mrs. Pine, age sixty-five, who had suffered a debilitating stroke.

Mrs. Pine cried often for no apparent reason. The R.N. explained that crying jags were common with stroke patients and nothing to worry about. Mrs. Pine had limited movement due to partial paralysis and atrophied muscles, and she could not speak. She was also incontinent, and changing her "diaper" would be one of my duties. With my briefing over, the R.N. sent me off to meet my new client.

I found Mrs. Pine sitting alone in her room, propped up by pillows in a large chair, facing the open doorway to the hall. Not much of a view, I mused. No wonder she cries. She wasn't crying then, though—to my relief, because I didn't have a clue how I would handle the situation. Looking at the lovely lady, I sent up a silent prayer: *Please let this go smoothly.*

Smiling, I leaned down so that my face was parallel with Mrs. Pine's and covered her hand with mine. "Good morning, Mrs. Pine. My name is Carol, and I'll be looking after you for the next three weeks."

Mrs. Pine didn't answer, but her face softened and her blue eyes watched me intently.

My duties the next morning included giving Mrs. Pine a sponge bath. When I removed the soiled Depends (I refused to call them "diapers" as most of the staff did. Talk about eroding a resident's self-esteem, I'd thought.), I was taken aback by the red marks on her buttocks. I reported the abrasions to the head nurse, and she followed me to the room and instructed me to gingerly apply ointment to the inflamed area.

"Does that feel better?" I asked Mrs. Pine.

Her eyes brightened, and she smiled.

So, this is what it's about—caring for people who can't take care of themselves, I thought as I washed my hands in the sink.

Mrs. Pine's smile faded fast, though, when I tried to dress her. Every time I took out an item of clothing, she would burst into tears and it would take several minutes to calm her down again. Aside from the inexplicable bouts of crying, we had no problems. Still, I could sometimes sense her distress, even when it didn't result in tears, and none of my ministrations seemed to relieve her discomfort completely or for long.

By week's end, I'd settled in quite well. I was performing my duties well, and I was enjoying the work. Helping to make the residents' lives a little easier gave me a feeling of purpose and satisfaction, and I was feeling more confident about my decision to change careers. One thing that continued to nag me, though, was feeling that I wasn't doing enough for Mrs. Pine.

During my weekend off, I couldn't stop thinking about Mrs. Pine. Though she was unable to speak or gesture, it seemed as though she was trying to communicate with her eyes, and I was sure she understood what I was saying. I felt strongly that the crying was due to her frustration with feeling helpless and not being able to communicate.

On Monday morning, I told Mrs. Pine that whenever she needed to go to the bathroom and I was within eye-shot, whether in her room or in the common areas of the center, to raise her hand and wave. She nodded and smiled. Within the hour, her arm was stretched high and her eyes were bright with excitement. I hurried over and pushed her wheelchair into the bathroom. Her Depends was dry, and as I helped her onto the toilet and she relieved herself, her excitement grew to laughter.

Wow! She isn't incontinent; she just needs someone to take her to the bathroom.

Mrs. Pine kept smiling and nodding her head, as if to say, *Yes, you're getting it! Yes, I can do this! Yes, please help me to do this little thing for myself, to retain my dignity.* I hugged her and promised to keep my eye out for her raised hand.

During report, I proudly told the head nurse about the incident.

"Well," she sniffed, "we don't have enough staff and enough time to cater to each resident."

Undeterred, I found the time, and Mrs. Pine continued to signal me when she had to use the restroom. And she cried less.

One morning I was down on my knees sifting through Mrs. Pine's closet when the head nurse walked into the room.

"What on Earth are you doing, Carol?" she barked.

"I'm trying to find Mrs. Pine's slippers."

Mrs. Pine had kept pointing at her feet and then at the floor and then at the closet, and after several guesses, I'd finally figured out what she wanted. She was very pleased when I retrieved them from the closet and patted my head in appreciation as I put them on her feet.

That evening at home I kept fretting about Mrs. Pine. *How can I communicate with Mrs. Pine? There must be a way for her to tell me what she wants and needs.* Then an idea floated into my mind. It was, shall we say, out of the ordinary, and "Bea Arthur" would probably have a conniption, but it was worth a try. I retrieved an old Spiegel catalogue from my bookshelf and ran upstairs to my office for a large sheet of cardboard, glue, and scissors. As I flipped through the catalogue pages and clipped and pasted, I wondered why I hadn't thought of this sooner. I just knew it would work.

The next morning I slipped into Mrs. Pine's room while she was eating breakfast in the dining room and hid the poster behind the table next to her bed. After her sponge bath, I asked her if the reason she cried was because she was frustrated.

She placed her head in the palms of her hands, and then looked up and nodded.

"That's what I thought," I said. "Mrs. Pine, I have a surprise for you."

I pulled out the poster, covered with pictures of clothing of all types and every color—dresses, sweaters, blouses, undergarments, nightgowns, slippers, shoes—and showed it to her, explaining how she could use the poster to tell me what she wanted to wear. Her eyes widened, and she clapped her hands.

For the rest of my three weeks as Mrs. Pine's nurse's aid, each morning and each evening, I would hold the poster in front of her and she would point to the article of clothing and the color she wanted. Her disposition improved tremendously; she seemed happier and cried less.

On the last day of my practicum, Mrs. Pine's family came to visit. They questioned what had happened to create such a change in her attitude. The head nurse asked me to tell them. After I explained about the poster, Mrs. Pine's daughter, Jean, hugged me so tightly I could hardly breathe.

"Thank you for doing that. Mother isn't as frustrated as she used to be," she said. "The nurse tells me she's also giving signals when she has to go to the bathroom."

Mrs. Pine grabbed my hand and squeezed it. That squeeze told me all I needed to know: that she was grateful for the small improvements in her daily life . . . that a little love goes a long way . . . and that I had made the right career choice.

Carol Sharpe

Providence

Her license plate always bothered me. Every time I swung into her driveway to pick up my son, I sat gripping the steering wheel, gazing at the neat house and pretty flower beds, the grubby basketballs and metallic bicycles littering the yard—anything to avoid seeing the back plate of the blue minivan parked in the driveway. *Lydia V*, it called out every time I dared to look. I'd wince and twist my neck to avoid the sight and memory of that name.

The van with the "Lydia V" plates belonged to Nada, the mother of my oldest son's best buddy. I first laid eyes on the license plate at the preschool where our sons had met on a sun-filled morning eight years earlier. Nada and I also met that day, when our spirited sons became instant and inseparable friends. I was immediately drawn to Nada's twinkling eyes and gentle smile. Her mismatched plaid outfit and white socks warmed her unpretentious chatter as she whispered to me about our sons, building with Legos together in the corner. Her words were tinged with an accent I could not place; I would later learn she had been born in Croatia and had emigrated first to Canada, then to the Chicago suburbs.

Her husband worked night and day, leaving Nada the brunt of raising three boys. At baseball practices, our vans idled side by side as we compared our lists of the day's activities, competing over which of us had more places to drive. I never heard a word of complaint in her sweet, calm voice as she shuttled the boys to sports, cello lessons, family visits, play dates, and doctor appointments. I did not meet her husband for three years. I teased her often about this, accusing her of faking a husband. To this she would softly laugh and invite me and my uncontrollable toddlers into her home.

"I love all the noise and the little ones here. It's too quiet without children's voices around," she would say. "Stay for dinner with us."

Nada busied her hands in the kitchen, tempting everyone with the smell of homemade sausage. Her welcoming home opened its doors to my family, and she embraced my son as one of her own.

I envied her quiet motherly radiance and devotion. Yet, occasionally, I detected a note of sadness in her eyes. She sat in church alone every Sunday, her smile turned pensive, no husband or sons in the seats next to her. Alone at the dusty baseball fields, she slouched in her folding chair, reading the Bible. Once I interrupted her reading, and I saw mist in her eyes as she tucked her Bible into her purse.

"It helps me when I'm having a bad day," was all she would say.

I assumed the sadness was loneliness, induced by her invisible husband, but I never pressed her to talk about it.

Nada's Bible always sat in the living room of her home, with its walls overflowing with family photographs. I traced her boys at each successive step of life, sprouting through the years in the photos, and I studied pictures of nieces, nephews, and Nada's family in Croatia. Never have I known someone who more purely and clearly revered God, valued family, and loved children than my friend Nada. Her appreciation of life's simple blessings humbled me. I always left her home and her company feeling peaceful and comforted . . . until I'd spot that license plate, "Lydia V," with its cold reminder otherwise.

The name "Lydia V" had haunted me for almost twelve years, since one September afternoon, when, as an inexperienced nurse, I answered the emergency room radio. My shift was over and I was headed out the door, my purse slung over my shoulder, when I heard the radio crackle. Paramedics were radioing a report of a six-year-old child struck by a car that had passed a stopped school bus. Their frantic voices forced me to grab the radio and start the preparations for the child, apparently critically injured. The evening nurses clustered around the radio, clutching their stethoscopes in silence.

Three rooms of the emergency department rapidly cleared, and the ER doctor became too quiet, his face taut as the nurses bustled in preparation. The veins near his temples bulged out as his face flushed. He shoved open the back doors of the emergency room and ran out to the ambulance bay, biting his lower lip. His daughter, Elaine, was seven. The day nurses stayed; we all looked around trying to ready ourselves in every way possible. Two nurses dragged over the square red pediatric emergency cart and snapped off the seal. While they fumbled with equipment, I flipped on the monitors, waiting for the green blips to come to life. Watching the second hand move on the wall clock, I tilted my head slightly to one side. In the distance, I heard the whine of sirens.

The paramedics burst through the doors with a cherub-faced little girl with golden hair, unconscious, her stomach rapidly swelling and exposed. Twelve pairs of hands attached monitors and tubes, each nurse attuned to every bark of the doctor's commands. We worked swiftly, crowding around the cart, calling her name over and over: "Lydia . . . Lydia . . . Lydia."

A Cup of Comfort for Nurses ⌐ 207

I clung to her side, holding her hand, and trying to get any type of response. "Lydia! Lydia, squeeze my hand! Do you hear us, Lydia?"

Throughout the entire half hour we frantically worked on her, the emergency room echoed with cries of her name. "Lydia" . . . "Lydia" . . . "Lydia."

Her parents arrived and tried to break past the police blocking the entrance door. Gently the police caught her mother, who wore a colored scarf wrapped around her head, as she crumpled to the floor. As Lydia's mother and father were led to an empty grieving room, our paths nearly crossed in the narrow entrance, but I turned away from her pleading eyes. A new nurse, I was distraught by the child's dire condition, the thought of her chubby cheeks and small hands now growing pale, and I knew her mother would see it in my eyes.

Lydia needed surgery, and as the operating room nurses pulled her cart away from us, I grabbed Lydia's hand and ran with her as they rolled the cart down the green hall into surgery with the only thought in my mind, *Don't let her die alone.* I was not then a mother. I had never seen a child die. But something inside me told me, *Stay with her. Hold her hand. Call her name.*

Lydia died in surgery, very quickly and quietly. To my disgust, I avoided her parents' eyes as I left. I wanted to tell them I had stayed with their little girl until the end, holding her hand, whispering loving words into her ear, but I said nothing. I drove home on autopilot and went straight to the bedroom of my tiny apartment. I fell on my bed and stared for hours at the ugly orange-flowered wallpaper, filled with guilt for avoiding Lydia's devastated parents. As a nurse, it was my job to comfort them, and because I'd allowed my own emotions to get in the way, I'd missed my only chance to tell them how sorry I was for their loss, and that their little girl had not died alone. I was numb with shock and shame, and my aching heart waited for tears that would not come. From that day on, I have carried the spirit of Lydia and her parents within me. Throughout my following years as an emergency room nurse, I have never again hesitated to reach out to others.

On a recent stopover at Nada's home to claim my son, I wandered past her photo wall and was drawn to the picture of a chubby-faced little girl with an impish smile, whom I assumed to be a niece or cousin.

"Who is this?" I asked my son's friend.

"Oh, that's Lydia, my sister. She died a long time ago. She got hit by a car."

I closed my eyes and reached out gently to touch her picture, not a breath left in me. My friend Nada, sweet Nada, was the mother of Lydia V.

Nada's laughter floated down the hallway, and I turned to see her squatting in front of my five- and six-year-old children, her face radiant. I felt a peaceful release inside me. Nada had given my children and me so much love and comfort over the years. Now I had the opportunity to give her the comfort of knowing that her child's last connection with this world had been holding a hand filled with love.

Mary Walsh Morello, R.N.

That Special Touch

I pulled my knitting a little closer to the light pooling across the hospital bed. The baby afghan was an old, familiar pattern, just something to keep me busy while I waited. I hadn't noticed daylight fading, but now shadows lurked in the corners of the room. They lurked in my mind, too. *What was taking so long?* I walked to the windows and stared out at the darkening city.

The orthopedic surgeon at home had hesitated to operate, because my husband's blood pressure tended to spike dangerously high when he was under stress. He warned us that a stroke could result. So, we had come here to the Mayo Clinic, 200 miles from home. I hadn't wanted to go to such a huge place. We knew our way around the hospital at home; here, I was sure we'd be lost within the first hour. Everyone had been so kind and helpful, though, and each nurse we met went out of her way to make us comfortable. It was almost like talking with the nurses back home.

An hour earlier, a young nurse with blond hair had come in to tell me that the surgery had gone well, but Bill would have to stay in the recovery room a while longer because his blood pressure was "a little elevated."

Would this result in the stroke we had been warned about? I worried. I paced from window to window, watching the lights of the cars flashing by in the twilight five floors below. I couldn't sit still and knit; I had to move.

A new nurse came in. She must have just come on duty. She had the softest brown eyes, and the hand she placed on my shoulder was warm and comforting somehow. Her name tag read "Marie."

"Have you had dinner, Mrs. Thatcher?" she asked.

I shook my head. "I'm really not hungry, and I expect my husband will be back soon."

"No. They just called. His blood pressure is still higher than they'd like. You go ahead downstairs and get something to eat. If he comes back before you do, I'll page you in the cafeteria." She patted my shoulder and nudged me toward the door.

The hot soup was good, and I relaxed a little as I chatted with two other ladies whose husbands were recovering from surgery. Even then, there lurked in the back of my mind the knowledge that Bill's blood pressure was still too high. I had prayed that the surgery would give him more use of his arm. The pain the last several months, the inactivity and inability to do all the things he loved—gardening, fishing, canoeing—and the hope that surgery would relieve all that, had brought us here. If he had a stroke now, he probably wouldn't be able to do those things anyway.

I couldn't stay away any longer and returned to my vigil by the empty bed. Surely he would be back soon.

Marie came in. Again the soft touch on my shoulder, the warm voice. "Mr. Thatcher will be here shortly. You ought to think about getting some rest, too. What time does the last shuttle come from your hotel?"

"In about an hour, at nine-thirty," I replied.

Shortly, the surgeon came in and gave me his assurances that all was well. Soon after he left, two orderlies wheeled in a gurney with my sleeping husband, and I gave God thanks for letting me hold his hand once more.

Marie came in from time to time to check on Bill and to encourage me to leave, always with a smile and a warm touch.

I sat by the bed for a long time, holding my husband's hand, my knitting abandoned, a puddle of pinks and greens on the chair. It was quite dark outside now, with very little traffic passing by the hospital. It was time for me to go, but the shuttle service was no longer running. I was looking in the telephone book for the number of a taxi service when Marie came through the door once more.

"It's eleven o'clock, Mrs. Thatcher. I have some reports to do, but if you could wait a while, I'll take you to your hotel on my way home."

I couldn't believe my ears. After working all day, she was volunteering to drive me to the hotel. Of course, I said I would wait as long as it took. We left the hospital at midnight. In the twenty-minute drive to the hotel, Marie chatted about the hospital and assured me that Bill would get the best of care and that she knew he would be fine.

Pulling up in front of the hotel, she said, "I'll just wait right here until I see you are safely inside the lobby."

I tried to thank her for her kindness but couldn't really convey how grateful I was. With a wave of her hand, she disappeared down the drive.

I never saw Marie again. She wasn't on duty the next day, and I was involved in learning the therapy that would be required when Bill went home. I never knew her last name, and I almost began to believe she had been an angel sent to help me. In time, I realized she was "just" a nurse, doing her job in her own wonderful fashion, with her very special touch.

Barbara Thatcher

Here's Looking at You!

I could never be a nurse. I know I don't have what it takes to deal with all that pain and suffering, and touching of boo-boos and bandages, and cleaning up people's bodily secretions, and hustling and bustling around on my feet for hours at a time.

My dad was a surgeon, so I grew up knowing that nurses were his eyes and ears, his data collectors and interpreters, and his hands-on helpers. I know he relied on them to relay every nuance of his patients, like who'd had a restless night and who wouldn't complain when in pain. I also knew how much my father respected the nurses he worked with.

I didn't inherit my dad's caregiver gene and I didn't follow him into the medical profession. Because I have an aversion to sickness and injury, and because I am a natural-born talker, I pursued a career in public relations. But wouldn't it figure that my first job was working in the public affairs office of the Medical College of Georgia. Part of my job involved interviewing researchers, doctors, and nurses, and writing about their responsibilities and contributions. The more I learned the more in awe I was of the whole medical profession. The researchers conducted research so the doctors could give the latest treatments, and the doctors worked long and hard to diagnose and treat patients. But it was the nurses who provided the main connection with and the main source of comfort to patients. It wasn't until later in my life, when I no longer worked within the medical field in any capacity, that I came to fully appreciate the true extent and value of nursing professionals.

When I got married, I traded in my briefcase for a diaper bag. Two children, a couple of moves to different cities and states, and a few years later, I decided to change careers and became a preschool music teacher. I've always loved kids, having fun, and singing, so it was a good fit for my personality. I collected and wore goofy earrings because I knew the kids would get a kick out of them. When I sang songs about peanut butter and jelly, for example, I wore peanut earrings. If our musical theme was about the spring, I wore bumblebee earrings one day and tulip earrings the next. My husband often joked that if I ever became a "civilian" again, I'd have no normal jewelry to wear.

After I had worked at the school for six years, my husband was transferred, once again, and it was time for another move to another state. The teachers chipped in and bought me a pair of gold hoop earrings.

The note inside their farewell card read, "Here's a normal pair of earrings to wear when you move. The people in the new town won't understand you at first."

When we relocated yet again, we ended up back where we had started, in the Augusta, Georgia, area. By then, my children were ten and twelve, and I was "just a mom" who took a few writing classes now and then. We were a very active, extraordinarily happy family. My husband and I loved each other, we loved our kids, and we loved our busy life. Then, in the midst of all that busyness, time stopped for us.

I was having some minor medical problems, which led me to go to our general practitioner for a routine checkup on a Monday morning. By Tuesday, our world had changed. I had chronic myelogenous leukemia. The only possible cure was to have a bone-marrow transplant. Our busyness went from shuttling children to soccer games and gymnastics to driving to countless medical appointments I'd rather not have gone to.

After months of hoping and praying and waiting, the time came for us to go to Emory Hospital in Atlanta for my bone-marrow transplant. My younger sister was the donor, a perfect match. In the Emory bone-marrow unit, every patient is paired with a nurse for each shift.

Those three main nurses would be my primary caregivers throughout my stay. They would do things for me that I normally wouldn't ask anyone to do. When I couldn't get out of bed, they would be my arms and feet. When I was hurting, they would be my pain control. When I felt hopeless, they would be my encouragers. When I behaved horribly, they would remain my patient, conscientious helpers. When I was happy, they would be the gracious recipients. When I was barely hanging on, they would be my rope and pulley.

Getting along with my nurses was at the forefront of my mind when I checked in on that windy Sunday in February. I prayed for someone who would be the nursing equivalent of my soul mate, a nurse I knew would have my back during this very rough patch. I asked God for a sign that He had heard my gluttony of prayers.

At 7:30 Monday morning, I met Diane, my primary day nurse. She was small, not much bigger than I am, perky, chatty, and efficient, completely on top of things. From her ears dangled two eyeball earrings. The next day she wore dice earrings, and the day after, something equally offbeat. During my entire two-month stay at the hospital, she never wore the same earrings twice and never once sported a "normal" pair. We were a match made in goofy-earring heaven, and from the moment Diane walked into my room, I was sure my prayers had been answered. I liked this nurse God had handpicked just for me.

Since I was on morphine and other mind-numbing medications much of the time, I often didn't know what was going on. So, what I'm about to tell you comes secondhand, as my husband relayed it to me once I'd returned to Earth from wherever I'd been, out there in my own private la-la land.

It was March 17, Saint Patrick's Day, but the luck of the Irish was certainly not with me. Everything went wrong. I had developed a yeast infection in my blood. The doctors called my family in from Oklahoma; I was in bad shape and declining fast. My parents came. My children came. My weary husband, who had been there all along, was beside himself; he didn't know what to do. Apparently, neither did the doctors.

That's when Diane took over. The doctors were standing around my bed discussing the options. Diane ushered them outside, and my husband followed them out into the hall, where Diane told the doctors in no uncertain terms not to discuss any uncertainty around me. She was aware that I was close to the breaking point. She suggested, strongly, that they come together with a secure plan.

After an intense consultation—outside my room, this time—the doctors ordered that my Hickman catheter be removed (believing it was responsible for my infection) and asked Diane to perform sixteen pic sights for my medications to be administered through. She said that she didn't think I could take all those sticks and suggested a central line in my neck. The doctors agreed with her suggestions. The procedure was performed, the problem was resolved, and my spirits were renewed.

My thirty-eighth birthday was just three days away. Thanks to Diane, on March 20, I got a little bit older. My daughter and son made a chocolate chip pound cake and brought it to the hospital for my celebration. I had not eaten solid food in weeks, and whatever bland thing I tried to eat just came right back up. But the mother DNA kicked in, and not wanting to hurt my children's feelings, I carved off a respectable hunk of cake and ate every bite . . . and kept it all down. Miracle? Or willpower? Who knows? I was just glad to be there, forcing down an extremely rich dessert, listening to my children sing "Happy Birthday," and living one more day.

Ten years later, I am relatively healthy and cancer-free. Words cannot adequately express my gratitude for all the things Diane and the other nurses did for me. Besides, I was so out of it during so much of that time I don't even remember half of it. What I do remember and will never forget is that the first day I met my nurse, she wore eyeball earrings. That's when I knew I would be okay, because I knew God had sent Diane especially to watch over me.

Jenny Lou Jones

Nurse Radar

D o you know why Miss Taylor is coming in today?" I asked Gayle, our trusty office coordinator, pointing to the third appointment on my schedule book.

Gayle had kept things running smoothly at the Green County Women's Health Clinic for years. Through the years I had come to count on her uncanny patient perceptions; she had a real knack for hearing what was left unsaid.

Her sparkly blue eyes fogged with worry. "She was vague about the reason for wanting to come in. But she was clear about wanting to see you. She asked specifically for Dana."

I had seen Sara Taylor a few times, but only for her annual gynecological exam, never for anything else. She was twenty-six years young, and aside from being painfully timid and mouse quiet (which initially led me to assess, then later to dismiss, clinical depression), she always appeared quite healthy. It had been only a few months since her last visit, and I wondered what could be wrong.

Before entering the exam room, I briefly reviewed Sara's chart. Four years of notes, all in my own loopy scrawl, revealed nothing I didn't already know. Her last visit had been three months ago to the day, and the pap screening had come back normal.

Perched on the edge of the white paper sheet that stretched across the exam table, Sara reminded me of the squirrels outside my kitchen window, always ready to dart and take cover in a flash. Her slender frame nearly evaporated beneath the sterile gown draped over her nakedness. Her limp, dishwater-blond bangs fell over one eye as she made an attempt to shift her gaze, without moving her head, from the floor to the door.

I have always been an outgoing gal who could easily carry on a conversation with a cardboard cutout, and I tended to think of such tight-lipped, introverted types as a mystery and a challenge. *Why could she make eye contact with the doorframe and not with me? What hopes, fantasies, or secrets might lurk beneath her hushed, taut exterior?*

"Hello there, Miss Taylor," I said. "I trust your school year is off to a good start. Are you still teaching second grade? Or did you switch to fourth this year? I seem to remember you mentioning that last time you were in."

She nodded, head still drooped, staring at her bony knees sticking out from under the paper gown.

"Fourth grade, that is such a great age; they're like little sponges then, aren't they?"

Again, she nodded, not looking up.

"And what brings you in today?" I asked.

Her eyes shot up and toward the door, then to me, and then back to the door, like a frightened mouse looking for an escape route. Finally her gaze settled on some safe spot midway across the collection of framed nurse practitioner licenses and the medical school diplomas on the wall behind me.

Her words came in spurts: "Well, um, uh . . . well, I've been having this, um, uh . . . itching, um, uh . . . and it's hot and, uh, stings when I use the bathroom. . . . I've never had it before. . . . But I've seen commercials . . . And my sister's had it, and she told me to grab some over-the-counter stuff at the drugstore. . . . But I wasn't sure . . . so, um . . . well . . . so, I guess . . . I'm wondering if you think I have a yeast infection." Her lavender eyes actually connected with my brown ones at the exact moment the question emerged. Just as quickly, she averted her glance—and was now scrutinizing the squiggly triangle shapes splattered across her medical gown.

While yeast infections are common in women her age, something seemed awry. It might sound odd, but one of my favorite parts of being a nurse practitioner is playing medical sleuth. I thrill to the challenge of gathering information and juxtaposing facts to figure out what is really going on with my patient, and so how best to help them. Over the years, I have acquired an internal detection system that picks up suspicious signals like some sort of nurse radar. Now, a very loud *ding-ding-ding-ding* was going off inside my head.

Senses heightened, I proceeded. "I'll need to ask a few questions, examine you, and possibly run some tests to determine what's going on. Okay?"

She nodded mechanically.

Gentle as rain, I sprinkled her with the necessary questions while completing the exam. I was simply following protocol, attempting to rule things out, and was shocked and disturbed as her answers revealed symptoms consistent with a sexually transmitted disease (STD). Her prim and proper presentation made it difficult to contemplate, but in an effort to be thorough, I felt obligated to pose tough, intimate queries. Clearly uncomfortable with my line of questioning, she gave one- and two-word answers in a phone-operator monotone. I listened intently, not only to her words, but also to her overall demeanor. Her stiff posture, trembling sighs, and total lack of eye contact were all crucial nonverbal clues. It was awful seeing her so distraught, but as much as I wanted not to make her uncomfortable, I knew that doing my job meant getting the information required to accurately diagnose the problem.

By the time she had returned to the safety of baggy pleated khakis and a plain white shirt, I had samples for the lab and had gleaned that she had had her first serious boyfriend and lost her virginity during the past year. She told me that she had had only one other sexual partner and that both had always used a condom.

"It doesn't look like a yeast infection, Sara."

She gulped, clutched together her white-knuckled hands, and asked, "What then?"

"We won't know for sure until the lab work comes back. Come in then, and we'll go over the lab results together."

Two weeks later, I found her in the only exam room in our office that is even somewhat cozy. Both she and her turtleneck were muted gray. She had selected the chair facing the wall. As I closed the door behind me, she closed *People* magazine, setting the entourage of this year's "best dressed" faceup on the table beside her. I took the chair across from her.

"Good morning, Sara. I hope you haven't been waiting long," I said.

"Not really," she said as she wrung her hands.

I decided to forego the tiny talk and get right to the matter at hand. Sara needed to know what she was dealing with.

After taking a deep breath, I said, "Sara, the results indicate you have syphilis."

I watched closely as a brief shudder of revulsion flickered across her face before she recomposed her blank expression.

"Could the test results be false-positive?" she asked.

"Not likely," I said. "When we receive reactive syphilis results, we double-check with something called a titer. The titer measures antibodies in your blood, the presence of which verifies the syphilis result. We also use a titer to monitor the progress of treatment."

Sara said nothing. She just stared at the floor, lost in thought or, perhaps, her own private hell.

"Sara?" I asked gently, and waited until she looked at me. "You appear to be in the latent stage of syphilis, which means you may have been infected a long time ago. When you first contracted it, you probably experienced flulike symptoms and maybe a rash. It is possible for syphilis—"

She cringed when I said that word.

"To remain dormant for years before the symptoms reappear. It is crucial that we figure out how you were infected and when," I explained. "The last time you were here, you told me that you had not been sexually active prior to last year. Is that correct?"

"Yes, that's right," she said.

I was watching her closely and got a weird vibe as her expression changed, briefly and almost imperceptibly, from one of confusion to comprehension.

"At this stage, the prognosis is good. Treatment will involve regular shots of antibiotics. We'll watch your titers," I said.

Now for the part I was dreading. Collecting myself, I continued, "I am required to report syphilis cases to the health department. Both of your previous male partners will need to complete a screening."

She squirmed, but remained silent.

"The nurse will be in to give you your first injection in a few minutes. You should also schedule another appointment in four weeks. Okay?"

"Okay," she whispered.

I thought of her frequently during that time, trying to fit together all the pieces. When the results for her sexual partners came back from the lab, I was both surprised and not surprised. On a dreary winter day, I informed Sara that both of her partners' test results had been negative. Her sigh of relief was followed by a tight-lipped grimace.

I reached across the table to hold her hand and ever so gently asked, "Sara, this isn't easy, but I have to ask: Were you sexually abused as a child?"

I felt her grip tighten and watched as she raised her eyes, looking directly at me for the first time. "From the age of eight until I was twelve, my grandfather had sex with me." She paused a moment, squeezing my hand and meeting my eyes. "I have never told anyone this before."

Sara cried then.

I wanted to hold her little eight-year-old self, and I wished I could have protected her from the whirling world of pain and fear that had been her childhood. Instead, I searched for words that might help the young woman heal her wounded soul now.

"Sara, you have incredible strength. What a devastating thing you have been through, and how hard it must have been for you to keep this inside yourself so long. I am very proud of you for sharing this with me today."

Quiet tears tumbled from her eyes.

"Where is your grandfather now?" I asked.

"He died. Severe dementia. Years ago."

I nodded, knowing that, left untreated, syphilis leads to dementia.

I stood and stepped to her side, and offered her a long, safe embrace. I held her tiny frame, wanting to absorb her suffering. As we moved apart, I saw gratitude and a glimmer of hope in her eyes. Perhaps now that her horrible secret was no longer walled up inside of her, true healing could begin, both in her body and spirit.

Resuming the role of plainclothes medical professional, I reviewed the treatment plan, explaining that she would need to get shots regularly, based on the volume of antibodies in her blood. I encouraged her to call a counselor for therapy and provided several referrals.

Sara followed my advice and began the road to recovery. With aggressive antibiotic treatment, the syphilis has gradually cleared up. Sara has also confided in me about her progress in therapy, and has blossomed into a vibrant young woman. The once-reserved Sara now has a playful glow in her eyes and a sweet, joyful smile. As her titers have improved, so, too, has Sara's self-esteem.

On her last visit to receive her antibiotic injection, Sara wore a fuchsia sweater, shiny hoop earrings, and mascara. Standing tall and looking directly into my eyes, she said, "Dana, because of you, I have been freed from this horrible secret. Thank you."

Grinning, I gave her a quick hug and said, "You're welcome, Miz Sunshine."

Then I grabbed the chart for my next patient and glanced through the intake notes:

Age: 37. Presenting symptoms: Eleven-month history of chronic fatigue, "hurting all over," sleeps poorly/wakes unrested, exhaustion increasing.

Hmmm . . . .

Yes, indeed, another case for Nurse Radar. I opened the door and strode confidently into the exam room.

"Hello, Mrs. Reed. Nice to see you again. So, tell me, what brings you here this fine spring day?"

Robin O'Neal Matson, as told by
Diane Kissel Burket, C.N.P.

Triumph in Trauma Room One

I t began like any other night in our rural hospital emergency room. We were suturing lacerations, nebulizing asthmatics, and x-raying baseball injuries when he was rolled into trauma room one. He was nineteen years old, he had curly blond hair, and his injuries were catastrophic. His truck had been hit by a train, and he was dying. I'm pretty sure he never knew anything that happened after the impact that night. I'm also pretty sure I will never forget it.

I had been an R.N. for many years and was well acquainted with tragedy. ER nurses learn quickly to compartmentalize their feelings; otherwise, they won't last long. But as I went out to meet his gurney being rushed in by the paramedics, my heart began to pound in my chest. That head of hair looked just like my little brother's. Frantically, I dug through his effects, looking for his identification; his first name was the same as my brother's. Why is it that a sudden shock can make your whole world reel? Why is it that my eyes took in the entire name, yet only the first name screamed inside my head?

The patient was not my brother, but in that instant, he became my family in a surreal way. I wanted desperately to save him. So did the entire emergency medical team.

We worked for hours. I think we all knew from the beginning that it was futile. But his youth and the savagery of metal upon flesh propelled us to use every miracle of human technology in our desperate attempts to forestall the inevitable.

While we feverishly sought to save his life, clerks sought to locate his family. Word filtered back to us that the father was home recuperating from open-heart surgery. He had sisters. The family was now in the waiting room.

The young resident and the experienced physician overseeing the code finally stepped back. "Enough."

The room was a disaster: blood pooling everywhere, cardiac monitor paper spilling over machinery, IV bags hanging from every available surface. The room was still and somber. Noticeably absent were the usual joking and bantering, attempts to break the tension. We were all shaken by the brutality of death and by our inability to arrest it. We were all overwhelmed by the reminder of our own mortality.

Any one of us, any of our loved ones, could be here one instant and gone the next.

I feel strongly that bodies need to be viewed, that families need to see with their own eyes that the best of care has been given and that their loved ones are truly gone. I believe that people who have lost someone suddenly and tragically need this closure. Yet, this time, I was just as sure that it was better for this family to wait until the funeral home had done their part.

I went with the physician to tell his family. They were huddled on the vinyl sofa in the waiting room— father, mother, and two sisters. We advised them to wait until he'd been cleaned up to see him. The father agreed; he did not want to see his son mangled. But his mother needed to see him immediately. So did his sisters.

We led them to the room. His battered face was toward the door, and upon opening it, his sisters screamed and fell to the floor in horror. I was unprepared for the response of his mother. She whispered softly, "Oh, my poor baby," as she moved across the room and gathered her son into her arms. She did not weep; she did not recoil. She held him, rocked him, and told him goodbye.

Instinctively, I knew this was a holy moment. I also knew I should leave, but I could not. I was mesmerized by what I saw, and I was healed by it.

I also knew that we, the wise and experienced professionals who had fought so fiercely to save this woman's son, had made a mistake in assuming that death was the victor that night. We were wrong to believe that this young man's life rested solely in our hands and that when our best efforts failed, all was lost. Something much greater was at work in trauma room one that night, and what remained in the wake of our lost battle against death was something more healing than medical technology and clinical skill could ever be—love.

That night, a mother's love transcended the death of her only son. That night, a mother's unwavering love for her child brought healing not only to her and her family, but also to those of us who felt defeated by our inability to stave off death. That night, love triumphed over death.

I am a better nurse because of that experience. It taught me that victory is not measured by lives saved but by lives loved. That strength is not calculated by the weight lifted but by the weight endured. That my value as a nurse is not determined merely by my skills and knowledge, but also, ultimately, by my compassion.

Sherrie Kulwicki, R.N.

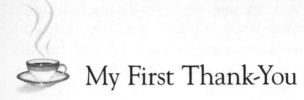

My First Thank-You

"How can you stand being a nurse? I could never do it; the smell of puke makes me want to barf." I can't count the number of times I have heard some version of this commentary, usually accompanied by a wrinkled nose and a look of disgust.

As a nursing student, I, too, sometimes wondered how I would be able to deal with the vomit, blood, and guts that nurses routinely face. But I didn't dare express my qualms in the classroom or when observing procedures or while doing my practicum with patients. Any such quibbling was sure to trigger a stern lecture from Miss Jo Horton, our pediatric nursing instructor:

> *If you're thinking of yourself, you're not thinking of the patient. How dare you give a moment's notice to the fact that vomitus made*

> *you want to puke, too? Think about how the poor patient feels. What can you, as the puking patient's nurse, do to make him feel better? Place a cool cloth on his head or neck, and clean up the mess. Assess his needs. Is he still puking, or does he feel better now that his body has rejected the indigestible foods? Perhaps a medicine has made him sick? Is there a need to call the doctor? Does he need nausea medication? And don't forget to write your findings in the chart. Remember, if it isn't documented, it didn't happen.*

Yes, I'd been on the receiving end of the "think of the patient, not yourself" lecture. I just never had the opportunity to put it into practice . . . until Miss Horton assigned me to an adorable toddler in the children's hospital.

Mikey had wavy blond hair and dark brown eyes. He also had a congenital defect called esophageal atresia, in which his esophagus ended in a blind pouch instead of connecting to his stomach. Since shortly after his birth, he had been fed through a surgically placed tube above and to the left of his belly button, directly into his stomach. At fourteen months old, Mikey was in the hospital recovering from surgery to reconstruct his digestive system so that he could eat normally, without the tube. Mikey could now chew and swallow food just like any other kid, and it went right to his stomach where it was supposed to go, instead of hitting a dead end. Except that his new digestive system wasn't quite sure what to do with food, and that's where I came in.

Mikey had just finished eating scrambled eggs, grits, orange juice, and milk. He obviously liked the new experience of eating and had eaten a tremendous amount. This big gob of food had rested in his grumpy stomach just long enough to get thoroughly acidified. I walked into the room to find Mikey sitting in the middle of his crib, erupting like a volcano. Volumes of yellowish soured grits, eggs, orange juice, and curdled milk gushed out of his little round mouth and ran down his hospital gown, all over his crib sheets, down between the crib bars, and onto the floor.

Gross, I thought, as I stepped forward. That's when it hit me: the smell. *Ugh!* I gagged convulsively, instinctively turning my head away and covering my mouth with my hand. I nearly added my breakfast to Mikey's. I didn't know what to do.

Nurse! I almost screamed out, but then remembered. *Oh, yeah . . . that's me.*

Willing my sense of smell to the lowest possible level, I took a halting breath . . . and promptly gagged again. Mikey stared, his eyes wide with surprise. I caught a glimpse of Miss Horton coming down the hall, checking on her students like a mother hen.

I breathed a sigh of relief as she passed the room. *Had she heard me? Was she giving me a grace period to collect my wits before flunking me in Vomit 101?*

The fear that Miss Horton had heard me gagging and would be disappointed in me was greater than my visceral reaction to the enormous pile of puke surrounding the saucer-eyed tyke in the crib. *I must think of Mikey. I must get him cleaned up—and pronto.* I looked over at the little fellow, sitting there so innocently and trustingly, staring at me as if to say, *Hey, what's going on? You're the big person here; do something already.* His lips started to quiver, and I suspected crying wasn't far behind. *Take care of the patient. Think of Mikey, not yourself.*

I dampened a wash cloth at the sink, and washed his darling face, gently reassuring him that everything would be okay. He twisted and squirmed, trying to get away, while I untied his pukey hospital gown and dropped it in the crud on the floor. I gingerly lifted him out of the slippery mess and sat him on a towel on the countertop next to the sink. Carefully, I bathed his chubby little body, paying special attention to the drainage tube connected to the little bag around his waist. Then, I toweled him off, smoothed sweet baby lotion on his soft skin, and dressed him in fresh PJs.

"Now, isn't that better?" I cooed as I lifted him up and gave him a hug.

His lips curved into a wide smile when I put him in his rolling walker. As I fastened the safety strap, Mikey lifted his pudgy little hand to my face and patted my flushed cheek.

Mikey just thanked me! In his baby way, Mikey just thanked me. Wow. My first thank-you! That feels good.

The nursing task, however, was not yet done. The hospital's "total patient care" policy meant that it was my job to meet not only Mikey's personal needs, but also his environmental needs. In other words: clean up the kid and the mess. With my lips pressed tight against any involuntary upsurge from my digestive tract, I removed the gooey crib sheets and blankets, folding the wetness to the inside, and tossed the whole aromatic mess into the hamper. I cleaned the floor with hot soapy water. Then I scrubbed the crib and sprayed it with disinfectant, leaving it to air-dry so fresh linen could be applied.

Just as I finished, Miss Horton came into the room to check on me and my patient. She talked with Mikey first, eliciting his beautiful smile and a barrage of baby words. I admired the ease with which she interacted with him. Then she asked me how Mikey's morning had gone.

I spoke only the facts, saying that his stomach apparently wasn't ready for a full-course meal yet, because he had lost his breakfast. And yes, I would properly document the incident.

"Well, he looks fine now," Miss Horton said, smiling at the toddler, who was happily circling around her in the walker. She turned her glance to me. "And how are you doing?"

"Fine," I said hesitantly, caught off-guard by her question. Then, more confidently, "I'm doing fine, thank you."

"Good," she said. "C'mon, Mikey, let's go for a walk."

I watched as Miss Horton and Mikey made their way down the hall, smiling at his stubby legs pumping to make the walker go forward.

Yes, I thought. *I am going to be just fine. I was able to think of the patient instead of myself.* That lesson has stayed with me and guided me throughout my thirty-five years as a nurse.

Lucile C. Cason, R.N.

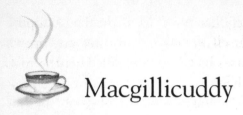# Macgillicuddy

Penny Starkey came home from fourth grade feeling unusually tired. Her mother put her to bed, where she slept until her brother called her to dinner. Dragging herself to the table, she sat silently as she watched her family devour her favorite meal— spaghetti and chocolate milk. She didn't have the strength to eat. She had less strength the next day, and the day after that her mother took her to the doctor. A barrage of tests revealed late-stage acute lymphocytic leukemia.

I met Penny the same day the doctors gave the grave news to her parents and admitted her to the unit where I worked. Despite the aggressive treatment plan, the outlook was grim. It would take a miracle to save her.

The hospital bed next to Penny's was occupied by a high school junior, Christine Sands—otherwise known as "Macgillicuddy." Christine had adopted the name for herself when she was three and one of the pediatric nurses had teasingly called her the nickname in much the same way other nurses called their patients "champ," "buddy," or "sweetheart." "Macgillicuddy" fit little Christine to a T, and it stuck.

Macgillicuddy was a frequent patient at Variety Children's Hospital in Miami, Florida, since her birth, due to osteogenesis imperfecta, a genetic disease of brittle bones that stunts growth. At sixteen, Macgillicuddy stood less than three feet tall—that is, if she could stand, which she could not. That doesn't mean she couldn't get around. She managed to do that surprisingly well by scooting and by rolling her manual wheelchair—a wheelchair that looked as though it were made for a doll.

Macgillicuddy bragged that she'd had more than 500 fractures. In a dresser drawer in her bedroom at home and in her locker at school were casting supplies. She'd learned to set her own bones when one snapped for no particular reason. On the day that little Penny Starkey was admitted to the hospital, Macgillicuddy was recovering from surgery she'd finally resorted to after her own doctoring had failed to stop the bone pain in her right leg. She was sitting in bed looking through a stack of brochures when I walked into the room to check on her and Penny.

"You look serious," I said. "Are you planning a trip?"

"No," she said, smiling. "I'm looking for art colleges that accept A-Ms as well as A-Bs."

"Oh. And what is an A-M?"

"Able mind. A-B means able body."

"I don't get it," I said.

"A-M . . . wheelchair accessible. There's one in Wisconsin."

"That's a long way from here."

"I know. That's the point. I want to get as far away from home as I can."

The statement shocked me. Macgillicuddy belonged to a close-knit, functional family.

"Why?" I asked.

"Because I want to be independent," she said. "Not like my sister who's going to the community college and living at home." Looking up at me she continued, eyes glistening with excitement. "I want to be on my own. You know, go to parties, football games, meet boys, join a sorority, stuff like that."

I'm not sure why that revelation surprised me; Macgillicuddy had always been independent. Here was a kid with a horrendous condition and acting as if it didn't exist. Though I admired her spunk, the thought of Macgillicuddy being away from her support system frightened me. She was so fragile. So vulnerable.

The next day Penny took a turn for the worst. While she endured a painful infusion of platelets, Macgillicuddy tried to comfort her.

"I'll bet you wish I was getting this treatment instead of you," she said.

"Oh, no," Penny said, looking at Macgillicuddy, "I don't want anybody to suffer like this."

Penny's words presented Macgillicuddy with a challenge. Later, after Penny fell asleep, Macgillicuddy pushed the nurse call light.

"Hey," I whispered. "What can I do for you?"

"Remember what Penny said . . . about not wanting anyone to suffer like she is? She's going to die isn't she?"

"Macgillicuddy, you know the rules about confidentiality."

"Sorry." She held tight to a brochure. "I wish I could be a nurse and help people the way you do."

My heart skipped a beat as I tried to think of something encouraging or at least intelligent to say. But all my mind could conjure up was how much of an A-M Macgillicuddy was. "I'm going to apply to this college in Boston." She handed me the brochure. "I think I can get a scholarship because of my grades . . . and my bones."

"A scholarship would be great. What happened to Wisconsin?"

"That school is liberal arts." Biting her lower lip, she breathed in heavily through her nose. "That one," she said, pointing to the brochure in my hand, "is more geared to sciences."

"Sciences?"

"Since I can't be a nurse . . . maybe I can do something . . . I don't know what exactly, but maybe social work or medical research."

"Knowing you," I said, smiling, "you'll do something to change the world and win a Pulitzer Prize on the way."

"I don't know about that, but it's time for me to be a little less self-centered." She glanced over at Penny. "Penny taught me that today."

"Penny is a strong little girl, and so are you," I said.

Later, I couldn't help wondering if Penny, by inspiring Macgillicuddy with her words, had fulfilled her purpose on Earth, because we never saw her ocean-blue eyes again.

Before Macgillicuddy had the chance to go to Boston, she won a scholarship to an art camp in Switzerland as one of ten promising high school artists in America. When she returned from that trip, she brought in photographs she'd taken of the majestic Swiss Alps to show the hospital staff.

"Where was this one taken?" I asked.

"We took a day off to go hiking."

"Hiking?"

Macgillicuddy smiled and shrugged. "There was this cute boy. My wheels can't hike, so I asked him to carry me piggyback. It was completely innocent."

"Imagine you off with some handsome guy in the Swiss Alps. . . . "

"And soon off to college!" she said, beaming.

Inspired by Penny's wish that no one should suffer, Macgillicuddy exchanged her dream of studying art for a different, more selfless dream. Instead of creating beauty on canvas, she decided to make the world a more beautiful place by becoming a medical researcher—hoping to ease human suffering and to give sick kids a chance to follow their own dreams. Because of her disability, she couldn't become a nurse, but she admired the values we practice and found a way to help those in greater need than she. Macgillicuddy made me proud to be a nurse.

Shelia Bolt Rudesill, R.N.

☕ Lady in Red

My decision to return to "hands-on" nursing was not made hastily or easily. The five years I'd spent as a coordinator for a provincial (state) home care program had provided a welcome respite from the physical and emotional demands of bedside nursing. But something was missing. The emphasis on fiscal responsibility made it increasingly difficult to provide the level of services clients needed. As a result, I felt like the connection I had with my clients was growing distant. A nagging voice kept telling me I wasn't where I should be, but I convinced myself that I was still making a difference, sitting in front of a computer, reaching out to people over the phone. Eventually, the voice of dissatisfaction screamed so loudly I had to listen, and I took a position as an R.N. in a geriatric unit, an area in which I had previous experience. My family and friends were baffled with my choice to return to working shifts, weekends, and holidays.

Reintegration has had its challenges. My skills needed updating, and I had to adjust to larger patient assignment and staffing shortages. I've also learned to swallow my pride and ask for assistance when faced with a new or difficult task, even those as simple as using a Hoyer Lift or the Vernacare, an archaic-looking contraption that disposes of bodily wastes. Reintegration has also had its upside. Instead of going home feeling empty, I go home exhausted but satisfied, hoping I made the right decision.

A few months into my new job, I still had lingering doubts about the wisdom of having returned to hands-on nursing. Sometimes, I felt like a fish out of water. Other times, the demands of the job made me wonder whether it was all worth it. Those uncertainties came to a head late one evening, deep into a long stretch of night shifts.

It was an exceptionally hectic night. Since the moon was far from being full, my coworkers joked lightheartedly that the vibrant red uniform I was wearing was having a rousing effect on the patients. We were busy answering call bells, resettling patients who were confused about their whereabouts, and providing medication for a variety of ailments. That alone would have kept us on our toes, but there was also Bert to contend with.

Bert was an emaciated, elderly man who was prone to aggressive behavior associated with his cognitive impairment. He seemed determined to spend the last of his remaining days yelling obscenities and pitching anything within his reach at whoever ventured into his room. Although Bert was often loud and disruptive, his feeble body posed little physical threat to staff.

At around 2:00 A.M., I cautiously peered into Bert's room to check on him. He was lying on his bed, covers strewn, rubbing his right ear.

"Get the hell outta here!" he yelled.

I scanned the bedside table for objects that could potentially take flight, and then cautiously entered the room.

"I said, Get the hell out of here!"

"I noticed you were rubbing your ear, Bert," I said calmly, ignoring his outburst. "Does your head ache?"

Bert had suffered from headaches most of his life, and the nursing staff was well aware that when he rubbed his ears, it usually meant he was in pain.

"Yeah, damn headaches. But don't try and give me any Tylenol. I'm not gonna take any Tylenol."

Bert eventually agreed to a warm drink. I helped him sit up on the side of the bed and sat with him as he slowly sipped the warm milk.

After a few minutes of light conversation, I sensed that he was actually enjoying the company. As I sat there listening to Bert ramble on about the time in his life when his body and mind weren't failing him, a sense of peace washed over me. The tensions and frustrations that had haunted me suddenly fell away.

When Bert had finished his milk and reverie, I resettled him back into bed and gently tucked the covers under his unshaven face. He closed his eyes and within minutes fell into a deep, restful sleep.

The next evening, when I peered into Bert's room, he was haphazardly making his way from the bathroom.

"How's everything tonight, Bert?" I asked.

He straightened slowly to acknowledge me, as I stood just outside his doorway in a crisp white uniform. Frowning, he looked me over, head to toe.

"Shit. I was hoping it was that lady in red," he muttered. "When is she coming back?"

She is back, I thought. *Right where she's supposed to be.*

Then, I smiled at Bert and cautiously walked into his room . . . carrying a glass of warm milk, fully prepared for flying objects and a bedside chat with a lonely, if surly, old man.

Dorothy Wright, R.N.

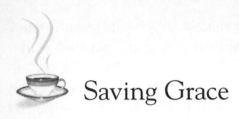

Saving Grace

While many Americans watched the Twin Towers in New York be destroyed the morning of September 11, 2001, I slept. Like most night-shift workers defying the body's natural circadian rhythms, I had difficulty getting sufficient rest. Despite dark curtains on my windows, I rarely slept well or enough. My family and friends, aware of my dismal sleep patterns, decided not to wake me until hours after the terrorist attacks.

When the phone rang at three, I stumbled to answer.

"Mom, the world is ending." I recognized my daughter's voice, but her comment made no sense. I pinched myself to make sure I wasn't dreaming.

"What are you talking about?"

"Mom, haven't you heard? We are under attack. Our country is under attack. Turn on the television."

Still gripping the phone, I headed for the television and watched in horror as the planes flew into the buildings.

"Mom? . . . Mom? . . . Are you still there?"

"Yes," I managed to get out, while I struggled to think of something to say to my daughter, hours away at college, that might reassure her that she, that we, would be all right when I, myself, couldn't get my fuzzy, confused brain around what in the hell was going on.

"When did this happen? How? Why? Why didn't you call?" The questions poured out of my mouth.

My daughter told me what little she knew.

"Can you believe that the university still held classes all day? I couldn't even think, so I just came home and watched the news. I was totally freaked out, but I didn't want to wake you."

In my disoriented state, it didn't immediately sink in that her concern for my health had taken precedence over her need for comfort as she'd watched the terror unfold on TV all day. My eyes glued to the unimaginable images replaying over and over on the screen, I realized I was failing in my parental duties at that moment, but I was speechless.

"You should be safe," I finally managed to get the words out. *But how could I know*, I questioned. *If people can fly planes into skyscrapers and the*

*Pentagon, how can I possibly know that anyone is safe,
anywhere, ever?*

"Do you work tonight?" she asked, jarring me back
to reality.

"I do." Still numb, I stared out the window at the
tall pines in the backyard. "I'd better get moving."

Any detailed memory of the time following that
phone call until I arrived at work is gone, overshad-
owed by the shocking destruction and loss of life
of the terror attacks. At some point I must have
called my son, who also was away at school, but I
can't remember anything we said. My husband and
I must have shared some sort of dinner; I doubt that
I cooked. Though I'm sure I showered and dressed
and drove to work, I have no recollection of having
done so.

At work, mood at report was somber. We were all
in shock.

In patients' rooms, the television news continued
to report the day's attacks. The death toll climbed
higher and higher; at one point it was estimated to
be more than five thousand. There was little chatting
and no joking among the staff. Though we performed
our duties as always and made a concerted effort to
be cordial and comforting to patients, we were clearly
subdued and distracted by the tragedy that had
taken place and that continued to be replayed and
rehashed on the news.

Then I was called to a delivery. A birth of an innocent child into what kind of world, I wondered.

As I scrubbed and gowned I tried to shake my dark thoughts, giving myself a pep talk. I told myself that babies were being born today, like any other day, all across the country, even in New York. I told myself that this baby, like those babies, would go home and grow up with families who would love and cherish them. I told myself that this child, all our children, would be all right.

But despite my best efforts to suppress my gloom, all I felt was sorrow for the defenseless child I was about to help deliver into a vile and violent world. *What's the point?* I thought sadly. My profession as a healer and facilitator of life suddenly seemed futile.

Then the routine of the job kicked in. Robotically, I prepared the bed warmer and also the emergency equipment and instruments, in case they were needed. The usual hustle surrounding a cesarean section prevailed. Somehow, I found the presence of mind to pray for a healthy baby and an uneventful delivery for the mother. Eighteen hours after terrorists took the lives of more than three thousand people, the newborn was placed on the warmer. No extraordinary pediatric medical assistance was required; only drying off the baby, administering the routine medicine, and wrapping the infant in warm, fresh blankets. A flawless delivery. A perfect, healthy infant. A happy, healthy mother. Still, sadness filled my heart, and thoughts of my country's losses preyed on my mind.

As the dad took his new daughter in his arms, someone asked what her name would be.

"Grace," he said.

Grace: mercy, goodwill, virtue, kindness, beauty of form and action, the spirit of God operating within humans to regenerate and strengthen the human spirit, a prayer of thanks.

As the baby's father spoke his newborn's name— "Grace"—I felt the shroud of despair lift from my soul. In that moment, I knew that our nation would heal and that our faith in the sanctity of life would be restored. Silently, I gave thanks for God's little messenger, whose timely birth on that tragic day reminded me that the job that has consumed much of my life—and deprived me of sleep—for more than thirty years is, indeed, God's work.

Linda Lee Hanson, R.T.

You Are the Nurse?

The day marked my fourth month in Belize. My husband and I had spent two weeks and shed buckets of sweat turning a dirty, dilapidated corner of a building into a medical clinic. Since then, I had spent long hours day after day attending to patients while geckos climbed the walls and termites built fresh trails on the ceiling over my exam table. Though I was a nurse, my duties had expanded beyond providing basic health care. I also disposed of the occasional dead rat on the path to the clinic, swept mounds of dead bugs from the floor, and waged daily war against mosquitoes big enough to ride. Once, I even armed myself with a machete and battled an opossum that wanted to make my clinic his home.

But on the day marking my fourth month in this tropical hellhole, I was taking a much-needed break from work. For one day, at least, I would be Nancy the Photographer and not Nancy the Nurse.

The pickup truck bumped down the winding road that would take us out to the countryside. In the pre-dawn darkness, the morning breeze felt refreshingly cool. I knew that the heat of the day would soon leave me drenched with my own perspiration. It was the dry season; although we passed towering fan palms and the thick understory beneath the towering trees of the rainforest, the road was parched and dusty.

The truck jerked along over deep ruts in the road as we made our way to the village. I had arranged to spend the day with a young woman named Terese, from whom I had bought a handwoven *jippa-jappa* basket a few weeks ago. Without a telephone or any other way to confirm our plans, I wondered whether my visit would be welcomed.

"Do you think she remembers? What if her family isn't as enthusiastic about my spending the day as Terese seemed to be?" I fretted to my husband as we neared the village. "You'd better stay at least until I make sure this is going to be all right."

As the truck lurched up to the small grass-thatched hut, I saw that my concerns were unwarranted. Terese and her entire family—all fifteen of them—were waiting by the road with wide smiles.

"Hello, Miss Nancy," Terese called out as I stepped from the truck. "I so happy you come. I so afraid you no come."

Turning to my husband, I grinned. "Fretting over nothing I see. See you back here before dark?"

"You bet. Enjoy your day off," he said. Then he disappeared back down the road, leaving a cloud of dust in his wake.

I had come to the village with an agenda: to play, not work. While nursing is my vocation, photography is my passion, and I was eager to capture the distinctive beauty and culture of Belize and its native people on film. I planned to spend the entire day, from dawn to dusk, photographing Terese and her family, with their permission, as they went about life in their Mayan home in the rainforest.

As they began their day, I observed and photographed the well-choreographed bustle of daily work. Most efforts involved food preparation for the midday meal, with all family members pitching in. I was amazed at both the rustic simplicity of their life and at how creative they had been in adding modern "technology" to lighten their workload. For example, to grind corn for tortillas, Terese has replaced the traditional flat rock and pestle with a hand-powered grinder much like the one my grandmother had used to grind meat. Terese boasted that her new grinder made her work much easier and faster; it now took only two hours to prepare the cornmeal and make the tortillas for lunch.

After the corn was ground, I helped Terese and her sister, Justina, gather the laundry and carry it down a dirt path to a small creek that ran behind their home. All ten little boys of the house, ranging in age from four to ten years old, accompanied us. On the way I tried to memorize their names and identify who were Terese's sons and who were Justina's. I learned that one of the children was actually Terese and Justina's brother. There were no technological advances for washing the clothes; just as their ancestors have done for hundreds of years, the women simply laid each piece on a flat rock, rubbed it vigorously with homemade soap, rinsed it in the creek, then wrung it out with their hands before placing it in a large handmade basket. Standing in thigh-deep water, Terese and Justina scrubbed each article of clothing carefully, taking great pride in how clean the clothes became.

Crouched like little monkeys, the boys lined the creek bank to watch the women. They seemed to be waiting for something to happen. When the laundry was done, the women walked out of the water and wrung their dripping skirts onto the ground. Terese nodded at the boys, and the frenzy began.

Peeling off their clothes, they jumped into the water. Laughing and shouting, "Watch me! Watch me!" they performed a show of underwater hand-stands, jumped from the creek bank over and over again, and swung from a rope tied to a tree high above, landing with a splash in the creek below. Such pure joy! I found myself laughing along with them, and I was tempted to peel off my clothes and join in the fray.

Soon, though, we headed back toward the house. There was more work to be done. The huge basket of clean laundry was carried back to the hut atop Terese's head, and then hung on the line to dry.

Next, Terese weeded the garden using a pointed stick and machete. "If we don't do every day, the forest will eat the garden," she explained.

While photographing the family going about their normal routines, I realized that everyone did his or her part with little or no discussion or instruction. They all seemed to know their respective role in the lively choreography of their daily life. Even the little boys returned after their morning swim to cut grass with sharp machetes. What had at first looked to me like the playful attacking of grass with their "weapons" soon turned to hard labor that caused tiny beads of perspiration to form on their little foreheads.

Later that afternoon we sat crouched on low stools outside the thatched hut in the shade of the cashew tree, resting and chatting. Occasionally, the soft afternoon sounds of a birdcall or cricket were heard. The morning work was over. Children were bathed; the laundry washed; the garden weeded; yams dug; corn ground; the tortillas cooked; the black hen killed, plucked, and boiled. We had filled our bellies with the simple food, and now was the peaceful time of day, the siesta, when the children played quietly and the women sat undisturbed, enjoying a few moments of female companionship and tranquility.

"You are the nurse?" Terese asked hesitantly.

"Yes," I answered, also hesitantly, reluctant to return to nurse mode just yet.

"For my sister—you have medicine to make no more babies?"

And so we talked. I learned that, at age twenty-four, Terese had four children and that her sister, Justina, twenty-six, was a mother of five. Both insisted they wanted "to make no more babies." They had many questions, which soon poured out. We talked. We laughed. We talked some more.

When Grandfather stepped outside the door to see why we were laughing, their talk quickly changed to the art of making jippa-jappa baskets. I appreciated that Grandfather was not to know their secret. Only when he re-entered the hut did our talk resume.

I felt like Margaret Sanger floating diaphragms into New York Harbor in whiskey barrels as I arranged for the women to walk ten kilometers to my clinic during their next moon time. They chose "the injection." They smiled. They sighed. They seemed so grateful, it more than made up for all those wretched mosquitoes, rats, termites, and opossums.

Today as I reflect back on that afternoon, so far away from home in a culture so unlike my own, I realize that my work is not a hat I can put on and take off. Even on holiday, I am the nurse. I also realize that in nursing, as with most things in life, it isn't the years and the things done that we remember, it is the people, the relationships, and the extraordinary moments. On that hot, dusty afternoon in a remote village in the middle of the rainforest, I shared such a memorable experience with two lovely young Mayan women. We talked. We laughed. We connected. It was one of my finest moments.

Nancy Leigh Harless, A.R.N.P.

The Stand-In

Some people would say I had spoiled her, but my youngest child, Jenna, would not go to sleep until I read her a story and rocked her until she got too drowsy to fight sleep any longer. The rocking was for me as much as it was for her, because after she was born, I was told I could have no more babies. My dream of having a large family was gone, and she would be the last baby I would have the joy of rocking.

When Jenna was about two and a half, she awoke one night screaming in pain. My husband, Joe, and I were too scared to wait until babysitting arrangements could be made, so we woke up our two boys and rushed to the hospital. A battery of tests revealed a large tumor pressing painfully inside one of Jenna's tiny kidneys. The doctors were amazed that it had not bothered her before. Joe and I took turns holding her, trying not to let our terror show, while emergency surgery was arranged.

For the first week that Jenna was in the hospital, I stayed with her day and night. The nurses put a rocker in her room so we could continue our nighttime routine. After she fell asleep, I got what rest I could in the stiff recliner that I scooted next to Jenna's bed.

Jenna was doing well, and Joe urged me to go home to get some decent rest and to spend some time with the boys, who, he reminded, needed me too. Also, the burden of his having to work full time and take care of the house and all the needs of the boys was beginning to wear him down. Reluctantly, I agreed that I should go home in the evening, have dinner with the boys, then return to the hospital until Jenna was asleep. Once she was down for the night, I would come home for the remainder of the night. The first time I saw the joy on my boys' faces when I tucked them into bed, I knew I had made the right decision. Still, I worried that Jenna would wake up in the middle of the night and cry for me.

Sleet began to fall one evening as I hurried home to make dinner. By the time our meal was done, the roads were treacherous. Joe stood by my elbow as I gazed out the kitchen window.

"I'm not going to let you out in this weather," he said firmly.

"Joe," I protested, "I have to read Jenna a story and rock her. She won't be able to sleep if I don't."

"Honey," he said, "be reasonable. What if you have a wreck and get hurt . . . or worse, and you are never able to rock her again?"

I called the hospital, unable to keep from weeping. "It's the first time since she was born that I haven't rocked her at bedtime," I told Sallie, the middle-aged nurse with bright red hair who worked the twelve-hour shift from 7:00 A.M. to 7:00 P.M.

"She'll be fine," Sallie reassured me. "I'll go in to see her before I leave and tell her that when she wakes up her mommy will be here."

"Thank you, Sallie," I said. "Tell her that I love her, too."

I woke up at dawn and was relieved to see that during the night the salt trucks had been by. Although far from being clear, the roads were in much better condition. I dressed hurriedly, certain that I would find Jenna red-eyed from crying for me. Remembering Joe's admonition from the night before, I forced myself to drive slowly.

I pushed open the door to Jenna's room, and my feet froze to the tiles and my jaw dropped. There, sitting in the rocker, was Sallie, snoring softly as she cuddled a peacefully sleeping Jenna. *The Gingerbread Man*, one of Jenna's favorite books, was lying on the floor where it must have slipped from Sallie's hand after she'd fallen asleep.

I tiptoed over and kissed Jenna softly on the cheek, then impulsively kissed Sallie too.

Sallie's eyes flew open. She blinked at me for a moment and then smiled sheepishly. "I didn't mean for you to catch me," she said.

"Sallie," I said, "your shift starts in an hour. How will you make it through the day?"

She smiled down at Jenna. "If I had walked away from her last night, I would have seen her little tear-streaked face all night." Sallie looked up at me, and I saw more kindness in those green eyes than I had ever seen in a human being before. "I can cope with losing a little sleep, but she wasn't coping very well with having to go to sleep without her mommy. Well, I'm not her mommy, but I think I was a pretty good stand-in. We rocked and read for a while, and both of us managed to get some sleep."

Before Jenna left the hospital, I took a picture of Sallie holding her in the rocking chair. The picture is in a frame on Jenna's dresser. I tell her often about the kind nurse who couldn't leave a crying little girl, even though her own family was waiting for her. Though Jenna is now six years old, she never tires of hearing the story. Last Christmas, she even named her new doll "Sallie."

I often overheard my grandmother saying that so-and-so was a "good person." It's an old-fashioned expression, but sometimes it is the only phrase that truly fits. Sallie is more than a good nurse; she is a good person.

Elizabeth Atwater

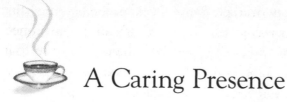

A Caring Presence

It is said that "nurses eat their young." Experienced nurses become impatient with the naive idealism of the eager novices. They sigh and shake their heads as they lament, "They'll learn soon enough about the stark realities of the nursing profession." New graduates enter a profession where patient acuity is high, staffing patterns are low, and discontent is the norm. Patients are stigmatized, and the caring ideal is challenged.

Seasoned nurses become hardened to death. In an era of high-tech medicine, death is seen as a failure, something to be avoided rather than assuaged. While miraculous cures are celebrated, the sanctity of death is obscured. People are reduced to objects, patients to clients. The necessary tasks of caring for the dying are performed quickly and often perfunctorily, to free time and resources for helping the living.

When a person dies, the focus immediately shifts to making room for the next occupant. No longer do nurses provide the reverent cleansing of the deceased's body; now, they call the funeral director to come and remove the cadaver as quickly as possible. Housekeeping efficiently cleans the room, and the nurse is ready for the next admission, hopefully someone who can be cured.

Nursing students have a more respectful attitude toward death. They have yet to fall into the routinization of patient care. For them, death is a fresh experience worthy of their time, care, and presence.

Though I can't remember all of the students I have educated over my many years of teaching, there are some I'll never forget. These are the novices whose untainted attitudes and idealism about their chosen profession informs not only my teaching but also my life. Laura was one of those students who taught me something about myself and my priorities.

Laura was a first-year student in my Fundamentals of Nursing clinical group. It is not easy for a first-year student to provide hands-on care in a skilled nursing facility. The patients have multiple illnesses and disabilities that require special beds, lifts, alarms, feeding tubes, and treatments. Many have difficulty speaking, and their bodies are ridden with contractures and paralysis. Some are dying. Making the transition from the mannequins of the nursing laboratory to the demands of a hectic clinical setting is a giant leap. Though Laura was understandably unsure of herself at first, she did well with her skills and showed unusual sensitivity to the emotional needs of her patients.

One day early on in her rotation, Laura heard of an elderly gentleman who was dying. Though not assigned to that patient, she wanted to observe his Cheyne-Stokes respirations, a symptom that death was imminent. Upon entering his room, Laura was troubled to discover that he was facing death alone. His family was not available, and the harried staff did not have time to sit with him in his final hours of life. The patient was unconscious, but Laura felt strongly that he needed a caring presence to ease his transition from life. She requested permission to stay with him as he died.

I am ashamed now of my hesitancy then, and of the objections that ran through my mind. He wasn't my concern. He wasn't assigned to my students. If the nurses on the unit don't have time for him, that is not my concern. I was busy with the task of educating students. I had important work to do. Besides, there was nothing to be done but wait for death to come. What would be the learning value in that?

I wanted to see Laura perform more important nursing skills: baths and dressings and transfers. I suggested this to Laura.

"No one should die alone," she said simply.

I knew in my heart that she was right. I compromised, telling her she could sit with him for an hour, but then she would have to return to her assigned patient. The time was 9:30.

Laura quickly searched the unit for a book and returned to the room with *Dances with Wolves*. To Mr. B.'s unresponsive form, Laura explained that she would stay with him until 10:30 and that she hoped he would enjoy the book. She pulled her chair close to the bedside, took hold of his hand, and began to read aloud in a quiet, soft voice.

Throughout the next hour, the other nurses and I would periodically peek into the room to see whether all was well. Laura never noticed; she was intent on reading. Her gentle murmuring could be heard as we hurried down the corridors, focused on our work. Laura's hand never let go of Mr. B.'s. His respirations eased into slow and shallow breaths. At 10:25, a fellow student looked in to discover that Mr. B. had taken his last breath. Laura was still reading.

After death had been verified, the primary nurse, Laura, another student, and I stood quietly around Mr. B.'s bed. The primary nurse said that you can often sense the moment when a person's spirit leaves his body. A few minutes later, we felt gooseflesh, a sense of release, and a sense of peace.

Some people believe that we choose our moment of death. I believe that Mr. B. chose to die in Laura's caring presence, hanging on until just before she was due to leave. I'm glad that she was able to see in her ingenuity what I had become oblivious to in my experience.

If only we could capture and preserve the idealistic perspective of our novice days in nursing. Perhaps then we would need no reminders that the work we do brings value to both the lives and deaths of human beings. Maybe then we would remember that nursing is not about inputs and outputs, reimbursements and profits, or risk management and accreditation. It is about helping to improve the quality of people's lives, every moment of life, with our caring presence.

Elizabeth-Ellen Hills Clark, R.N.

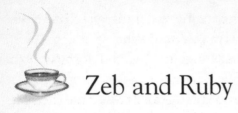 Zeb and Ruby

A rosy dawn illuminated the sky as I left home and headed for the hills. Fog lingered in deep hollers, waiting for the sunrise. Before the day was out, I'd cover a hundred miles, racing from one end of our big Appalachian county to another on my home health nursing rounds. I dreaded it, and drew no comfort from the glorious daybreak, took no mind of the wild beauty of Kentucky's mountains. I was too busy worrying about money and the pressing need for a new car. The year was 1995. By then, my nursing career had spanned decades. I was tired in mind and body, floundering to maintain a spirit of compassion and concern. That day, the anticipated peace of an early retirement repeatedly crossed my mind as I navigated the winding mountain roads. All I wanted was for that day to come and this day to end. To make matters worse, a new case had been added to my already jam-packed caseload.

I spent that first visit to Zeb and Ruby's cabin completing a thorough nursing assessment of Ruby. As I worked, a chipper and energetic Zeb told me their life story. He emphasized that they were ninety-one years old now and delighted with their lot in life.

They'd been starry-eyed teenagers when they "went to courtin'," in Ruby's words. As was the tradition in those isolated Kentucky mountains, Zeb built them a cabin from the ground up with his father's help. Trees growing on the home place were felled and split by hand, and then aged a season before the cabin was constructed. Zeb told me it was a "rough but tol'able" home for his bride and him to share. He considered the building of it, the hard work that went into it, a symbol of how much he loved his wife-to-be.

Seventy-five years had passed since Zeb and Ruby moved into that cabin in the holler. Their rough log home had weathered many seasons, but I imagined it still looked pretty much the same as it had three-quarters of a century ago. Zeb proudly pointed out how snugly the aged logs still fit together and the packed dirt floors Ruby swept each day. I looked around. The cabin's dark interior was lighted only by a coal oil lamp and daylight peeking through one tiny window. Their double bed took up one corner of the living area.

Its head and foot were hand-carved pine. A colorful hand-pieced star-pattern quilt covered the bed.

Ruby sat in a large leather chair Zeb had positioned a few feet away from the bed and fireplace. Big happy smiles lit up both their faces as I listened to Zeb's stories and checked Ruby's heart and lungs.

As if to reassure me, he said, "No drafts will ever blow on Ruby, and our floors are always clean."

I nodded my agreement with that statement while zipping up my nursing bag. Their home was cozy, and the dirt floors clean as polished rock. My modern, costly home came to mind as Zeb and Ruby waved goodbye.

I hadn't paid attention to the cabin's setting on arrival, but took in the surroundings as I left. Zeb said he had carefully chosen the site for their cabin. He'd wanted his new bride to be proud and happy with her home. A narrow dirt lane wound from their cabin through thick primeval hardwood forest. The woods provided deep shade in summer and protection from snow and penetrating wind in winter. Fragrant wood smoke rose from their field-stone chimney and lingered on the wind. I felt refreshed and energetic, and couldn't wait to visit them again.

I got to know Zeb and Ruby well in the course of my assignment as their home health nurse. It was a humbling experience. They were content with their lives and had no grand illusions about wealth or their position in society. Their primitive cabin had no running water or indoor plumbing, no TV, phone, or electricity. They got satisfaction from the unspoiled land around them and joy from simple blessings, and they still loved each other madly. Zeb said it best: "We can make do, the way we always have, together."

Neither one could read on more than a rudimentary level, but they were proud that they'd learned to write "enough to get by." They'd raised several children in their two-room cabin. Ruby did their massive washings by hand and hung clothes out to dry on a line strung between two oak trees. She still cooked on the same wood-burning stove Zeb had bought her as a wedding present. Zeb farmed on a small scale, plowing with mules, raising corn and huge amounts of vegetables that Ruby canned to feed their family. They'd never had the luxury of indoor plumbing, but Zeb assured me that their ice-cold well water was pure and free of taint. Every conversation was sprinkled with humor and their gratitude at having such a long and joyful life.

Zeb's eyes twinkled proudly the day I asked if I could take their picture. He said I could but only if the fireplace was included and he could hold the Kentucky walking stick he'd whittled nearly fifty years ago. The fireplace had always been the center, the heart, of their home. He'd made it himself of native stone and cast iron. It had warmed them all their married life. That day, its burning coals put out a soft warmth as I helped Zeb and Ruby pose their chairs close to the hearth. Carefully, Zeb arranged their favorite treasures on the mantel before he took his seat and smiled in preparation for the picture. Between them, on the mantel, sat a small glass paperweight shaped like an owl, a fist-size pink quartz rock he'd found while plowing, and a small oak-framed print of Sallman's "Head of Christ."

Their three elderly sons stood off to one side while I snapped several pictures. All lived nearby on the same home place and had gathered in special celebration of the day. Ruby's need for home health services had ended. Because Zeb and Ruby considered my last day as their nurse a memorable event, they "paid me honor," as they called it. Ruby baked an impressive tin of biscuits and made a cast-iron pot full of sweet cream gravy. The biscuit pan she'd used all their married life, which was nearly three feet long, was filled with soft biscuits done to a golden turn. She'd made the gravy with homemade sausage, bacon drippings, flour, and milk from their own Jersey cow.

Zeb said a prayer of thanks before our meal was served, then somberly presented me with my own plate. "This is a plate of honor. No one will ever eat from it again," he said. "After you've gone, Ruby will wash your plate and fork, and then I'll sit them on the mantel. Each time we look at your plate, we'll remember you and smile."

That simple, kind gesture touched my heart, and I couldn't stop the sudden flow of tears that came when Zeb handed me my plate. Well, we all ate too much of Ruby's good cooking that day. Zeb groaned and rubbed his stomach, saying, "I've et until I foundered!" For another hour or so, we laughed at Zeb's tall tales and smiled at his tender flirting with his ninety-one-year-old sweetheart.

I visited Zeb and Ruby as a friend many times after that day. Zeb made a little wooden frame for the photograph I'd taken of them and sat it on their fireplace mantel. During the two months that I was Zeb and Ruby's nurse and their friend, we exchanged life stories, shared humor and hope, and forged a deep and lasting connection between us. Knowing them taught me that open-hearted humanity should always be my focus as a nurse.

During my forty-year career as a registered nurse, many patients have faded fast from memory, while others have brought new perspectives to my role as a caregiver. Zeb and Ruby are both gone now, but their impact on every aspect of my life continues to comfort and encourage when my spirits flag and the realities of our modern world seem overwhelming. The lessons I learned in their old Kentucky cabin are with me always, guiding and giving richer meaning to my work and life.

Laurel A. Johnson, R.N. (retired)

Relinquishing a Soul

I watched a stranger's heart beating today. It was the size of a fist, flesh-colored, and pulsating as blood pumped oxygen through his vascular system. I knew little about the man whose naked body lay before me, only that he had come into the emergency department four days earlier as a hit-and-run victim with a closed head injury, two fractured femurs, multiple broken ribs, and a fractured right arm.

One of the surgeons asked if I wanted to observe the procurement of organs. I thought about the recipients, somewhere, waiting for the delivery of a kidney or a liver. *Were they dreaming of organs, packed tightly in ice, flown to their destination, to be transplanted in their failing bodies?* I wondered if their thoughts weren't mixed with the sadness of losing a life to gain a life.

This was something new to me, as I worked in the postanesthesia unit and seldom ventured into the operating rooms. I hadn't viewed a surgical procedure for years and had never seen a beating human heart.

Two masked surgeons were gowned and gloved while one nurse filled out paperwork and the other set up suction and positioned the overhead lights. A surgical tech gathered shiny steel instruments and formed the sterile field around the patient.

The body on the gurney had been ventilated for the past four days. Callused areas appeared on his feet and hands. He was a large, muscular man, thirty-five years old, with a mole the size of a dime on his left hip. When I leaned in close over the gurney, I could see his pulse beating in the arteries of his neck. When I touched his arm, it felt warm and resilient, just like mine.

His family said he wanted to be an organ donor and assist others in need when he no longer had use for his body parts.

I watched as one of the nurses prepped his upper chest with Betadine and the surgeons prepared to cut. The man's lateral chest was discolored with purple and red ecchymoses, and his broken arm was bandaged with cast padding and ace wrap.

The surgeon spread sterile towels that hid the patient's face, but from behind, I saw thick strands of his long, dark hair. Every few minutes my eyes wandered down to the coarse black hair that moved with the slightest motion. It somehow proved that a person was under the sterile blue cloths. I didn't want to see his face; that would have been difficult. It might remind me to look once again at the monitors that provided evidence of life—heart rhythm, heart rate, and oxygenation—proof that he was still living, not yet departed from our world.

The surgeon started to cut, as if unzipping a parka from the patient's lower abdomen up to the base of his neck. Then, with a sharp instrument, he sawed lengthwise so that the rib cage could be parted, before installing a large retractor that pulled the two sides of the incision apart. Now it was as wide as it was long.

Dressed in blue scrubs, a yellow isolation gown, and a mask, the surgeon held an electric cauterizing wand. It looked like a cheap bank pen on a cord but functioned like a scalpel. The wand cut and burned as the surgeon made his incisions, melting shut each severed vessel, causing less bleeding and an odor like seared meat.

Even on the inside, the patient looked very much alive. I watched the pulse of his heartbeat in his liver and all the way down to his aorta. The electronic beat from the heart monitor reinforced the impression that the patient was a living, breathing, thriving person.

I thought about my science class in high school and how I had dissected frogs. Some of the girls had giggled and turned red, but I'd wanted to take part in the dissection and learn about their anatomy. I used sharp blades to carve out organs and set them on a blue towel before labeling. I watched the delicate hands of squeamish girls unable to cut through the slimy skin. Boys laughed to cover up their feelings while slicing their frogs into cubes. The ambiguity I felt then was with me today.

In college, I remember the cats, all different sizes and colors, waiting to be dissected by eager prenursing students. Then there were the cadavers, a man and woman who donated their bodies to science so that nursing students could probe and use scalpels to dissect each organ. Somehow it seemed easier to work on bodies that were cold, stiff, and discolored than to observe organ procurement. I knew the cadavers were dead; more like rubber mannequins than humans, but the man on this gurney had soft skin, with some color to his face, and his symmetrical lungs moved up and down with equal breathing—inspiration and expiration.

An anesthesiologist stood behind the hidden face, watching the monitors and regulating the patient's oxygenation. The hum of the ventilator, the beats reverberating on the screen, and the click of the staple gun blended in with Billy Joel's greatest hits, playing on the stereo. I stepped up on a stool to view the opened chest and stared at the amazing muscle, the human heart, counting the beats and watching the synchronized movement gently lift and fall. It's a mixing-machine part, the human body's most animated organ.

The patient had hepatitis C, and transplanting his heart was not an option. But his kidneys and liver would benefit a needy donor.

I watched as the surgeons carefully examined his liver, turning it from side to side and noting the healthy color and size. They said it would be sent to California for a hepatitis C recipient. One of the donor network nurses explained that people with hepatitis C share the same body chemistry, and so a recipient with hepatitis C adapts easily to a hepatitis C donor's kidneys and liver.

I stared at this brilliant creation, thinking about God's creatures and my heart, your heart, the hearts of all the staff in the room. I've heard that when surgeons take out a heart for transplant, the room becomes silent, prayerlike. They say that once you hold the human heart in your hands, you'll understand that feeling. It's like holding someone's soul.

The lungs were striped with black lines from smoking, and I wondered what those tar-damaged organs might have looked like in thirty years. The intestines were as long and amazing as I remembered them, a coiled labyrinth of machinery perfected by the same Creator. One of the surgeons bundled them together under sterile green towels, as they continued to suction and do their work.

The abdominal and thoracic aorta had to be cross-clamped before the kidneys and liver could be removed. I watched as the heart muscle quieted, as the fast dance became a slow waltz. It quivered a bit before it stopped its movement. The anesthesiologist turned off the monitor and the ventilator and left the room. His work was finished.

A dose of Heparin was given to prevent clotting, as a nurse poured crushed ice into the abdominal cavity. The surgeons suctioned out blood before procuring the liver and kidneys.

The differences between life and death became issues in my mind as I tried to understand the organ-donation process. I thought about the spirit and soul and wondered what the difference was. I'd always felt the soul to be in one's heart. I wanted to pinpoint the precise moment when the spirit, the soul, whatever you wish to call it, has ceased to exist. This very body that looked only bruised an hour ago began to turn a darker shade with a tint of blue and had a hardened, cold exterior. I knew the look of death. Before my eyes, the body had discernibly altered. Something—call it spirit, or soul, or life force—had departed. I heard myself sigh deeply, as though, with his departure, I too had been freed. The quandary of that thin line between life and death was no longer there.

I thought about a soul's passing. *Do departing spirits fly by loved ones, brushing against them in noticeable ways? Do they hover over their useless bodies, procrastinating over their fate?* I'd heard many stories. A patient in the recovery room told me she had once died in a previous surgery and was brought back to life.

"I was above my body, looking down at the chaos taking place in the surgical room. Then I was in the waiting room watching my husband and family cry in a corner. I knew the time wasn't right to die," she'd said. "When I recovered, my heart and soul were somehow changed. I saw things in people I never noticed before."

We looked at one another and held each other's hand. We both understood.

But this body lying before me wasn't going to recover. His soul and spirit must move on. *Is there a special heaven set aside for people who die like this?*

I listened to the sound of my own breathing, felt the puffs of breath that circulated around my blue mask. I breathed in and I breathed out. For a moment, I felt lost even within the area around me. I looked across the room and imagined all of us with that miraculous muscle pulsating, keeping us alive, that familiar sound reverberating in my ears when

I place my stethoscope on someone's chest: *lub-dub, lub-dub, lub-dub.* We were here, my coworkers and I, still part of the material world, our souls still somehow, somewhere attached to our bodies, perhaps to our hearts. Rays of light seemed to radiate through the room, past the man with long, dark hair, past the surgeons and nurses. And I knew a man's soul had moved on.

Terry Jean Ratner, R.N.

A Miracle for
Miss Mattie

As a charge nurse in a busy neonatal intensive care unit, I have had my share of highs and lows in caring for newborns with odds stacked against them. Never have I experienced more joy or sorrow than when a certain preemie made her disquieting entrance on February 7, 2004.

When the pager went off that gray February day, my high-risk neonatal team—a neonatologist, a respiratory therapist, another R.N., and I—headed for the delivery. When we arrived, the labor and delivery nurse gave us a quick report. The baby's condition was grave. With weak heart tones and infected amniotic fluid, she was being delivered by emergency cesarean section at only twenty-six weeks, fourteen weeks early. The mother was under a general anesthetic and could not give my team any sort of direction or guidance as to how much we should do to help her baby. The labor and delivery nurse also informed us that if the infant survived, and the chances of that were slim, she would most likely be given up for adoption. The mother had too many problems in her life to take on another child, much less a fragile preemie requiring extensive and special care.

The baby was delivered quickly. She was limp and had only a whisper of a heart rate as I placed her on the warming table. The team worked hard for fifteen minutes to bring her back. We tried everything in our protocols, but her heart just wouldn't respond. Her lungs were filled with the same infected fluid, and even her umbilical cord was falling apart from infection. We worried that being without oxygen for so long had damaged her brain and other vital organs. With nothing left to try, the respiratory therapist and I wrapped the baby in a warm blanket and gently washed her face. With tears in our eyes, each member of my team held her and told her goodbye.

There were no visitors waiting and the mother couldn't talk or move, so I made a silent promise to the baby that I would hold her and not leave her alone. The RT and I took her to a quiet room to wait for the mother to wake up in case she wanted to see her baby. I sat quietly with the baby and softly stroked her face, telling her it was okay to be an angel; her brothers and sisters needed a guardian angel. The labor and delivery nurses came by to see her and say goodbye.

As we sat and talked gently to the infant, we noticed that she was slowly getting pink. It took us a minute to realize what we were seeing. Then she opened her eyes as if to say hello. I unwrapped her and saw that she was very pink—and wiggling. I quickly placed my stethoscope on her itty-bitty chest and confirmed that her heart rate was up. We called the neonatologist back to help us make a decision on what to do and then wrapped the baby back up and took her over to the NICU.

In the NICU, the tiny baby girl—all one pound, nine ounces of her—caused quite a stir. Her vital signs were close to normal, but we knew that wouldn't last. We put her on a ventilator to help her small, immature lungs and put in IV lines for fluids. We even gave her a quick sponge bath to guard against infection. That first night we expected her to be unstable and to get worse, but she proved us wrong.

As expected, the mother had decided to give her up for adoption and chose not to see or name her. One of the nurses decided "our" baby needed a name and dubbed her "Matty," which means strong, courageous one. She even looked like a Matty. She had quite the attitude as well.

The next morning I stopped by to see Matty before my shift began. She had had a stable night and was doing well. I sat by her bedside, watching and talking to her. I was off the rest of the week, and called in several times to check on her, something I rarely do, but I couldn't resist this time. I was afraid an infection would take over and she wouldn't make it. I should have known better than to have so little faith in Miss Matty.

At the end of the second week, we received incredibly good news. A family had taken a leap of faith and decided to adopt Matty, fully aware of the potential consequences of her early delivery and rough start in life. When the family learned that the nurses had been calling the baby Matty, they knew instantly that this was their baby girl. They had tried for a while to have a baby, and if they ever had a girl, they had planned to name her "Mattie." Matty became Mattie, and her new parents waited anxiously for her to become healthy enough to go home.

Mattie's family came in every day for the three months she was with us. We all watched her grow in awe. Considering her rough start, Mattie had a surprisingly benign course. She managed to wean off the ventilator relatively quickly, and then to tolerate her feeds. She was content to just sleep and grow.

Today, Mattie is ten months old, healthy, and full of energy. She is meeting all her milestones, and to look at her now, no one would ever guess her story. She is a beautiful little redhead with the best smile.

Her adoption was final this fall, and her parents can't get enough of her. I keep in touch with them, as I feel a special bond with Mattie.

Mattie gave me something I really needed: hope. At the time, I was going through a difficult period. I was in the middle of a divorce, taking care of my two young sons alone and trying to help them understand and cope with the changes in our family; working in a high-stress job; and struggling to hold all the pieces together. The miracle of Miss Mattie showed me that with a little faith and a lot of love, anything is possible.

Now, every time I think of Miss Mattie, I am reminded of another miracle: the power of human touch. Those of us in the nursing profession must never forget that as valuable and vital as medical technology is, so too are the healing instruments of our hearts and hands.

Barbara F. Iffland, R.N.

The Last Dignity

I was on my way to lunch break when I heard her scream. The sound was unmistakable: the cry of someone in excruciating pain. My tuna sandwich and *Oprah* magazine could wait; I made a beeline for room 8 of the hospital emergency room where I worked as an R.N. Upon entering, I noted two striking and seemingly incongruent things about the patient standing there: her dignified appearance—flawless makeup, perfectly coifed hair, stylish clothes—and the look of anguish and desperation on her face.

Terri, another R.N. in our department, was the primary nurse for this patient, but I could see she needed assistance. The patient, too wracked with pain to sit and too weak to walk, needed to urinate but refused to use a bedpan or to have a Foley catheter inserted. Obviously, no one had explained to her that a Foley catheter is a simple, discreet, and temporary device meant to make her more comfortable.

Mrs. L. was a sixty-two-year-old grandmother who had received a terminal diagnosis just four weeks earlier; small-cell carcinoma of the left lung had metastasized to her kidneys and bones. The Duragesic she'd been prescribed for pain weeks before didn't begin to touch the pain she had awoken to that morning. Unable to walk or even to get out of bed, she had asked her hospice nurse to call 911.

I tried to coach Mrs. L. about the advantages of having a catheter inserted, but she insisted that the doctors send her home, and that was that. No more invasive procedures, no more heroic efforts, no more trying to forestall the inevitable. It was over, and she was done with it. She'd had enough.

"No dignity, just death," Mrs. L. said bitterly.

The effort of speaking caused her to tremble, and she grasped my hand for support. Being a jewelry lover, I couldn't help but notice her beautiful, colorful bracelets. She apparently loved the ocean and everything in it. Her bracelets featured dolphins, sea turtles, and seagulls. Softening a little, Mrs. L. explained that she didn't want to lie down on the examining table to use a bedpan or for a catheter, because she knew that once she did, there would be no getting up again. She pleaded with us to assist her in using the restroom, and I agreed to help.

I beckoned for an ER tech to bring a wheelchair, but Mrs. L. flatly refused. Sitting was even more painful than standing, and she was so weakened, both from the disease and from the unsuccessful chemotherapy and radiation she'd undergone previously, that the energy it would require her to sit and to get back up seemed onerous. It took us a good fifteen minutes to get her four feet across the hall. She grimaced and moaned with each step, her fragile legs barely strong enough to hold her own weight.

When we entered the tiny bathroom, Mrs. L. paused and looked directly into the mirror, her piercing blue eyes scrutinizing her ghostly parchment skin. Even the expertly applied makeup could not mask the aura of impending death that shadowed her once-lovely face. Terri, the other R.N., stood on one side of Mrs. L., and I stood on the other; in the confined space, our right shoulders brushed the tiled walls. With each of us bracing one of her elbows with one hand while we supported her back with our other hands and arms, we started to slowly and carefully ease her down toward the toilet seat. After only a few inches, she cried out in pain: "Stop!" There we held her, semisupine, as though suspended in air—unable to sit at a 45-degree angle, unable to relieve her bladder distention, unable to move any farther down or up.

Her daughter knocked lightly on the door. "Is everything okay?"

After making sure Terri had a tight grip on Mrs. L., I quickly opened the door and darted out. Forcing a calm smile, I nodded reassuringly at her daughter. I grabbed a #16 Foley catheter with an attachable leg bag and headed back to the restroom.

I knelt in front of the beautiful, proud woman, took her hand in mine, and looked directly, and with great compassion, into her face. As I quietly and respectfully held her gaze, the defiance smoldering in her eyes flickered and gave way to a somber acquiescence. With no words spoken, we'd made a pact that I was going to make this as dignified for her as possible. She began to sob. I gently squeezed her hand, my silent promise that, with her permission silently granted and her trust in me gained, I would now do my best to bring her this small comfort. She reached out to stroke my face, perhaps in gratitude. I knelt closer to the floor and asked the other nurse to lift Mrs. L. a little higher, and after quickly sterilizing the area, I inserted the catheter. Mrs. L. sighed as the pressure of her bladder released. I quickly attached the leg bag to the Foley catheter and spoke to her about the privacy and cleanliness the device offered.

We carefully adjusted Mrs. L.'s clothing to its proper position, aware that even the slightest movement increased her pain. We dried her tears and patted her face with a warm washcloth, and then we inched her up to a standing position. As we walked slowly across the hall, I complimented Mrs. L. on her lovely jewelry, especially the dolphin bracelet. It was a strand of platinum dolphins, each dolphin separated by a bright stone—ruby, topaz, and multitudes of others. She said that she'd always had an eye for beautiful things. Once back in room 8, Terri and I scooped up Mrs. L. and laid her as gently as possible on the nonemergency stretcher.

Mrs. L.'s daughter was relieved to see that her mother was more comfortable, and she thanked us for our "special effort." With nothing left to do but go over discharge instructions, which Terri had well in hand, and with only fifteen minutes of my lunch hour remaining, I said goodbye to Mrs. L., kissing her lightly on the cheek and stroking her face as she'd done mine, and then headed off to the cafeteria for my delayed lunch.

One busy afternoon a few weeks later, the hospital's patient representative called to tell me I had a visitor in the front lobby. It was Mrs. L.'s daughter, who greeted me with a warm hug and tears in her eyes. She told me that her mother had passed away and thanked me again for giving her such "special care." She presented me with a card from her mom, which Mrs. L. had inscribed a few days before her death. Inside the envelope was the spectacular dolphin bracelet I had admired. Also enclosed were two photographs. The first was recent, of a frail but dignified and still beautiful older woman—Mrs. L. The other photo was worn and frayed, but I could easily make out the stunning young woman in a crisp nursing uniform, with eyes so blue they pierced my soul. I hadn't known before then that Mrs. L. was a retired nurse, but somehow I was not surprised to learn that she was one of us.

Those forty-five minutes I spent providing a small measure of comfort to a dying woman might seem unworthy of such acknowledgment and gratitude. Bedpans and catheters are not, after all, among the more heroic and esteemed aspects of nursing. Indeed, much of the time, many of those in the nursing profession, myself included, perform these and other seemingly mundane tasks with little thought to the impact on the patient. We don't pause to ask ourselves, *How does it feel for a proud and once-vibrant woman to no longer be able to walk to the bathroom, sit on a toilet, or pee on her own?* As we go about the necessary task at hand, we don't often consider, *How can I get the job done while honoring the patient's wishes and preserving her dignity?*

On that one day with that one patient, I took the time and had the presence of mind to ask myself those questions and to respond accordingly. Perhaps because that patient happened to be a nurse, she recognized the rarity and the merit of that. Now, I wear her lovely dolphin bracelet as a daily reminder that my every action and interaction with each patient provides an opportunity to make a positive difference in that person's life. Because of that dignified woman with piercing blue eyes, I now know for sure that, as nurses, it is not only what we do but how we do it that matters.

Lisa Lemming-Morton, R.N.

The Least of These

A heavy wooden door separated the emergency department's waiting room from the triage office, but its thickness was not enough to hold back the foul odor coming from behind it. With no small measure of dread, the triage nurse opened the door and found a dirty, disheveled man in a wheelchair. She quickly learned that he had come that day seeking care for the sores on his legs, the source of the awful smell. With eyes lowered in shame, he confessed that he had frequently injected intravenous drugs into the veins of his legs, causing large, festering wounds.

There were many open rooms in the ER on that unusually quiet Saturday morning, but none of the nurses wanted this patient. When no one volunteered to be his nurse, they decided to draw lots to determine who would care for the man. The nurses put their names on tiny pieces of paper and asked the ward clerk to pick one from a rectangular plastic basin.

"How did I know it would be me?" the chosen nurse lamented.

Sighing, resigning herself to the task at hand, she walked to the waiting room, politely introduced herself to the man, and dutifully wheeled him to a treatment room in the ER.

The homemade dressings, which were merely strips of torn cloth, were crusted to the man's legs and required a great deal of soaking before they could be removed. The stench from the abscesses was nearly unbearable, yet the nurse went about her duty and chatted with the man as she worked.

She learned of how he had been thrown out of his girlfriend's apartment and had been sleeping on the streets. He spoke with sadness and humility, thanking the nurse each time she left the treatment room and apologizing for the condition he was in. The nurse was overwhelmed with compassion. She ordered the man a warm meal and covered him with clean blankets while he waited to be admitted to the hospital.

Several months later, as this same nurse was arriving to work, she was met by a neatly groomed man standing outside the emergency department's entrance. He stepped toward her as she approached the automatic door, and when she stopped, he addressed her.

"You don't remember me, do you?" he asked with a twinkle in his eyes.

She sheepishly confessed she did not.

"I'm Joe Smith. You took care of me when I had sore legs. You were very kind to me."

The nurse's eyes widened in surprise, recalling the wretched state the man had been in when she had last seen him. She did, indeed, remember, and looking more closely at his face, she was nothing short of amazed at the transformation. Not only was he healthy, but he also seemed happy and confident.

He smiled proudly. "I wanted you to know that I'm clean now, not doing any more drugs. And I wanted to say thank you for taking care of me."

To this day, I am ashamed of how repulsed I had been by Mr. Smith's condition that day in the ER and at how reluctant I had been to care for him. It makes me think of the stories in the Bible about Jesus touching and healing lepers. Although the unlovely are surely the hardest to love, they are the ones especially for whom we are called to care. It was a lesson I'll never forget—and one I believe the Lord wanted me to learn.

In fact, had I looked at every piece of paper in the "lottery" basin that quiet day in the ER, I wouldn't have been at all surprised to find my name on every one of them.

Barbara Loftus Boswell, R.N.

The Healing Art
of Friendship

I like velvet pillows, mashed potatoes, clouds, and long walks in botanical gardens. Their presence in my life brings comfort.

Nursing was a comforting part of my life, too, for close to forty years. Though I worked as a nurse for twenty-five of those years and have been "officially" out of nursing for the last fifteen, I have maintained my nursing license and still think of myself as a nurse. I resigned from my position as an R.N. because of a combination of factors. Like most experienced nurses, I was feeling wiped out and burned out. Also, and perhaps more important, I sensed it was time for a change. When I lost my parents in an automobile accident and received a small inheritance, I decided to take the opportunity to take some time off. I never went back to nursing. But does anyone ever really leave this profession?

This year I turned sixty. I wanted to mark this milepost in a special way, and a friend suggested I make it my "jubilee" year—a time of fruitfulness, harvest, and planting new seeds for future growth. I'm keeping a journal of my sixtieth year, and writing down my "jubilee" experiences has made me more aware of each day's blessings and joys. Some of my best jubilees this year have come from my renewed friendships with a group of nurse colleagues from my past. I reconnected with these nursing school class-mates about five years ago.

Having moved around a lot, I had been out of touch with my former classmates for many years. I was working in a religious bookstore, and one day a new customer, a woman about my age, asked me about a book she wanted to purchase for a physician friend's birthday. As our eyes met, we immediately recognized one another from thirty-four years earlier, when we had been close friends in nursing school. It seemed as though we were suspended in time, and the desert that my life had become was suddenly awash with flowers, like the pink, yellow, and coral blossoms that adorn cacti in the spring.

There was to be a "Class of '65" reunion soon, she said. Would I like to go?

Perhaps. . . . Yes. . . . But I was flat broke. Years of coping alone with the usual stresses of life as well as dealing with repressed memories of childhood trauma had drained my resources. I now felt more like the "client" of the nurse standing in front of me than her friend. My humanity hurt. Although a few threads of faith still held me together, it seemed fragile, easily blown here or there by even the slightest breeze of doubt or fear.

Another classmate paid for my trip to the reunion.

"I have been looking for you for so long!" she exclaimed. "Where were you?"

She also gave me a large check, shushing my objections.

"Here," she said. "This covers all the birthday gifts I couldn't give you when I didn't know where you were."

Her generosity moved me to tears, which came not in a trickle but in a torrent that mirrored the abundance of her compassion.

From that larger reunion, we have since branched off into a small, nurturing group of five nursing classmates who are now integral parts of each others' lives. There is me, of course, a desert flower in full bloom again, thanks, in part, to having reconnected with my nursing friends. My creative spirit and love of nature, and our silent vow to "be there" for one another, connect me with these "birds of a feather" just as our shared history as nurses did in our younger years.

One of us is a recent widow, planning to retire soon. This sweet and steady tower of strength has spent her entire nursing career in labor and delivery, helping mothers bring new life to the world.

Another of us just retired from years spent as a school nurse. Now she puts her nurturing spirit and helping hands to work in her church and community.

The third member of our close-knit group is a long-time cancer survivor, full of knowledge about holistic health and inspiring us with her joy in living. A henna rinse covers her gray hair, and her red-orange scarf flies behind her in the wind. She likes cats.

The last of us is a fairylike wisp who recently retired and emptied her nest. She is now preparing for the retirement of her physician husband. Though she no longer needs to be on duty for the early shift, she still rises at dawn for her full day, sipping her first cup of coffee at 5:30 A.M. Her heritage is Irish, and her husband's is Asian. Their home is a blend of East and West that is healing and expansive for the spirit—filled with music, art, and life and with myriad windows opening onto vistas of green, flowers, and frogs hopping in the pond. We other four are always welcome there, and often gather in that soul-soothing environment for easy companionship and laughter.

Though my classmates and I are now in the autumn and winter seasons of our lives, with our nursing careers behind us, we still find ourselves in the mode of being comforters and consolers, including with each other. We've developed a group sense of humor and often send one another funny little e-mails to brighten our days.

We've not only grown closer with age; we've also grown more alike. We all prefer noninvasive surgery now, and holistic meditation tapes provide gentle wisdom through our headphones. Our latent artistic bents are emerging—with art, music, writing, gardening, and cooking. We like strolling through museums and going to concerts. We volunteer for social causes and serve our churches and various community organizations. We still listen well when someone needs to talk.

During a brief conversation with a new friend some years ago, she suddenly asked, "Are you a nurse?"

"How did you know?" I asked.

"Because you tip your head, ever so slightly, when you listen to me. Nurses do that, you know."

One of my classmates has a lovely painting in her house of a young woman with her head tipped to one side. Maybe it is a painting of a nurse. My nursing friends and I often sit with our heads tipped toward one another, listening, sharing, strengthening, and comforting one another simply by being there.

In my days of bird watching at a local botanical garden, I learned that winter walks have a special beauty. After the leaves have fallen, the birds stand out against the barren landscape, and I can see the black-and-white chickadees, the scarlet cardinals, the orange-breasted robins, and the blue jays with a clarity not possible in other, greener seasons.

My classmates found me in a desert time of my life and watered my landscape with love, renewing my spirit and filling it with bouquets of sweetly scented flowers.

Nurses, I've found, are a deep well. Even after a full career of giving and caretaking, it is still possible to draw from that depth, over and over, to give to others. Having a nurse in one's life is a special gift—a jubilee of the highest order.

I still like velvet pillows, mashed potatoes, clouds, and long walks in botanical gardens. They bring me comfort. But I love the four nurses who have brought the comfort and joy of friendship to the autumn of my life.

Constance L. Gray, R.N. (retired)

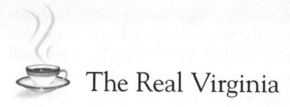

The Real Virginia

I was a new nursing supervisor when I met Virginia, a registered nurse who'd worked in labor and delivery for more than twenty-five years. Every day, Virginia came to work armed with two large shopping bags filled with catalogs, photos of her grandchildren, and anything else she felt she might need during her shift. Virginia was very tall, with broad shoulders and strong arms. Her size, coupled with the fact that she called me by only my last name, made her seem rather intimidating. I assumed her personality matched her rough exterior.

After watching her in action, though, I realized how wrong my first impression had been. Time and again I'd hear her voice from the labor room, gently and calmly reassuring a patient who was in pain, guiding her compassionately and expertly through the birthing process.

I often took my coffee breaks in Virginia's department, and if she wasn't busy, she'd sit and talk with me. I learned that she'd been raised by Polish-speaking parents, and she could speak the language fluently. Her husband had died young, leaving her to raise their ten children alone. She loved to dance and once had hopes of being a flamenco dancer. Instead, she entered the civilian nurse corps during World War II, taking advantage of the free tuition and a chance for an education that would enable her to support her family.

Virginia loved to tell stories about her experiences in the delivery room. One time she rushed back from her dinner break because a patient who spoke only Polish needed encouragement. Virginia rushed into the delivery room to find the patient was moaning with pain, and she immediately began whispering words of encouragement to her in Polish.

Suddenly, the patient stopped moaning, propped herself up on her elbow, and yelled in English, "Why is this nurse whispering gibberish in my ear?"

Apparently, Virginia had been directed to the wrong room.

Virginia also liked to talk about the "old days" in nursing. "We washed blood from the sheets ourselves before sending them to the laundry," she'd say. "Those were the days of rubber tubing and enamel enema pans." "I remember when we nurses helped to plant gardens on the hospital grounds to grow food for patients."

As time went on, I became quite fond of Virginia and the way she related to her patients. She was a patient advocate in the truest sense. She called things as she saw them and didn't take anything from anyone if a patient's well-being was at stake.

Five years after I met her, after more than twenty-five years of nursing, Virginia retired. On her last day of work, I noticed some security guards talking excitedly as a small crowd gathered in front of the hospital's main entrance. A white stretch limousine had just pulled up to the hospital's entrance. When the chauffeur opened the limo, out came Virginia with her shopping bags. Her kids had sent her to work in the limousine; at the end of her shift, the limo returned to take her home.

How fitting, I mused, thinking back to the day when I'd first met, and misjudged, Virginia. She was a skilled and dedicated nurse who had brought great compassion, humor, and style to her work. She deserved a stylish ride home from the place where she'd given so much with such class.

Joyce Franzen Kopecky, R.N.

This story was first published in *Nursing Journal*, June 1993.

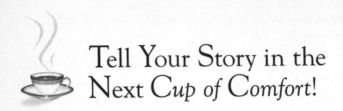

Tell Your Story in the Next *Cup of Comfort*!

We hope you have enjoyed *A Cup of Comfort for Nurses* and that you will share it with all the special people in your life.

You won't want to miss our newest heartwarming volumes, *A Cup of Comfort for Christians* and *A Cup of Comfort for Women in Love*. Look for these new books in your favorite bookstores soon!

We're brewing up lots of other *Cup of Comfort* books, each filled to the brim with true stories that will touch your heart and soothe your soul. The inspiring tales included in these collections are written by everyday men and women, and we would love to include one of your stories in an upcoming edition of *A Cup of Comfort*.

Do you have a powerful story about an experience that dramatically changed or enhanced your life? A compelling story that can stir our emotions, make us think, and bring us hope? An inspiring story that reveals lessons of humility within a vividly told tale? Tell us your story!

Each *Cup of Comfort* contributor will receive a monetary fee, author credit, and a complimentary copy of the book. Just e-mail your submission of 1,000 to 2,000 words (one story per e-mail; no attachments, please) to:

cupofcomfort@adamsmedia.com

Or, if e-mail is unavailable to you, send it to:

A Cup of Comfort
Adams Media
57 Littlefield Street
Avon, MA 02322

You can submit as many stories as you'd like, for whichever volumes you'd like. Make sure to include your name, address, and other contact information and indicate for which volume you'd like your story to be considered. We also welcome your suggestions or stories for new *Cup of Comfort* themes.

For more information, please visit our Web site: *www.cupofcomfort.com*.

We look forward to sharing many more soothing *Cups of Comfort* with you!

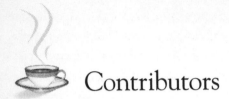

Contributors

Julie Alvin, R.N. ("The Lamplighter"), works as an obstetrics nurse at Good Samaritan Hospital in Downers Grove, Illinois. She lives in nearby Glen Ellyn with her husband, Dale, and their three teenage children.

Elizabeth Atwater ("The Stand-In") resides in Pfafftown, North Carolina, a lovely little town bursting with Southern charm. Though her primary job is being an adoring wife to her wonderful husband, Joe, she earns a living as a technician for Procter and Gamble. The second love of her life is writing.

Barbara Loftus Boswell, R.N. ("The Least of These"), lives in Aston, Pennsylvania, and works as a nurse manager at a crisis pregnancy center. She is involved in peer counseling and abstinence education. Her stories have appeared in two other anthologies.

Barbara Brady, R.N. ("Clarity in the Midst of Chaos"), is a retired recovery room and geriatric nurse, living in

Topeka, Kansas. She and her husband, Merris, have three children and eight grandchildren. She enjoys volunteer activities, writing, and most of all, family and friends. Her stories have been published in *Rocking Chair Reader* and other publications.

Karen Buley, R.N. ("Lessons from 3-West"), is an obstetrical nurse and writer. She has been published in *Family Circle* and in the *Missoulian*. She lives with her husband, Rich, and two sons, Eric and Colin, in Missoula, Montana.

Lucile C. Cason, R.N. ("My First Thank-You"), resides in Loganville, Georgia. She writes short stories and poetry, and is working on a novel about her many years of nursing experiences. Lucile's first published piece appeared in 2004, in *Small Town Life* magazine.

Jane Churchon, R.N. ("A Hazard of the Trade"), lives in Sacramento, California, where she works as a recovery-room nurse. The mother of two children, Jane writes in her spare time and also enjoys reading, travel, folk music, and a wide circle of friends.

Elizabeth-Ellen Hills Clark, R.N. ("A Caring Presence" and "Touched by a Student"), has taught psychiatric nursing at the University of Maine for twenty years, where she continues to learn from her students and patients. She lives in Hartland, Maine, with her husband, John, who is a writer and librarian. She has two grown daughters.

Maryellen Clark, R.N. ("On Borrowed Heritage"), is a home health nurse in the Blue Ridge Mountains of North Carolina.

Nan B. Clark ("When the Patient Is Your Mother") and her husband, Tom, both history buffs, founded an organization in their hometown of Beverly, Massachusetts, devoted to preserving an elegant nineteenth-century carriage barn on the grounds of President William Howard Taft's summer White House. She is a freelance writer.

Joanna Collie ("Inside the Caring Business") was born in Oxfordshire, England. She spent twenty years in Cape Town, South Africa, before settling in Leicestershire, England, as a radio writer, novelist, and intrepid local historian of small happenings that nobody's ever heard of.

Linda Swann Dumat, R.N. ("A Beacon in the Storm"), is a registered nurse who holds a bachelor of science degree in nursing from Vanderbilt University and a master's degree in adult mental health nursing from the University of Cincinnati. She is now retired from the Department of Veterans Affairs and private practice and resides in Tennessee.

Constance L. Gray, R.N. ("The Healing Art of Friendship"), of Bronx, New York, is a church administrative assistant and freelance writer. Her writing has appeared in a spirituality magazine and in a local newspaper. During the twenty-five years she was a nurse, she worked in a variety of specialties, including behavioral health, oncology, and addictions.

Shanna Bartlett Groves ("Scared, Healed, Delivered") is a Kansas-based writer whose work has appeared in *A Cup of Comfort for Sisters* and the *Kansas City Star*.

Linda Lee Hanson, R.T. ("Full Moon" and "Saving Grace"), has worked as a respiratory therapist in eight hospitals in four states over the past thirty years. Happily married for thirty-one years and the proud mother of two adult children, she is grateful for the coworkers and patients she has encountered, all of whom taught her about life and courage.

Nancy Leigh Harless, A.R.P.N. ("Over Coffee with Sister Filje" and "You Are the Nurse?"), is a nurse practitioner now exercising her menopausal zest through travel, volunteering in various health-care projects, and writing about those experiences. When at home, most of her writing is done in a towering maple tree, in the tree house built specifically for that purpose by her husband, Norm.

Marilyn J. Hathaway ("The Importance of Being Harold"), of Gallup, New Mexico, embraced hospital volunteering upon retiring from nursing and has served as president of local and New Mexico state auxiliaries. With her husband, she loves to visit their eight grandchildren and to travel, often writing while waiting in airports. A freelance writer of essays and devotionals, she publishes in magazines and anthologies.

Kathleen Herzig, R.N. ("My Amazing Shift with the Handsome Dude"), has spent most of her thirty-one years as a registered nurse working in critical care in hospitals in Ontario, Canada. She still finds "the bedside" a rich and privileged world, where she often receives so much more than she could ever give.

Barbara F. Iffland, R.N. ("A Miracle for Miss Mattie"), lives with her two young sons and two dogs in Idaho. She has been a neonatal nurse for thirteen years and enjoys all its rewards. She also enjoys reading, fishing, working in her yard, and playing with her kids.

Bonnie Jarvis-Lowe, R.N. ("Of Comrades and Comets"), of Newfoundland, Canada, began her thirty-four-year career in nursing in the operating room and then switched to bedside nursing. After retiring at age fifty-one, she has pursued writing and photography and enjoys outdoor recreation. At get-togethers with her three sisters, who are also nurses, nursing is often a topic of conversation.

Laurel A. Johnson, R.N. ("Zeb and Ruby"), is a Marysville, Kansas, native now living in Fairbury, Nebraska, with her husband of forty years. She recently retired from her long career as a registered nurse. She is the author of three published books and writes reviews for several online and literary journals.

Jenny Lou Jones ("Here's Looking at You!") lives in North Augusta, South Carolina, with her husband, Lance, and dog, Matlock. A creative writing workshop presenter in area schools, she also speaks to churches about how God held her in his hand as He led her through her survival of leukemia and a bone marrow transplant.

Sandy Keefe, R.N. ("My Brother's Keeper"), is the health-care manager at Camp Costanoan, a special-needs camp in Cupertino, California, devoted to providing meaningful outdoor experiences and socialization for children and adults with developmental disabilities and physical challenges. Her thirteen-year-old daughter Allie is a regular camper there.

Lyndell King ("A Double Dose of Courage"), following her student nursing experience, went on to pursue disparate fields and now lives in Tasmania, Australia, with a husband, two rambunctious homeschooled boys, and a variety of creatures. She recently completed her first novel.

Joyce Franzen Kopecky, R.N. ("The Real Virginia"), has three loves in her life: family, nursing, and writing. She spent the last twelve of her thirty-five years in nursing as an evening supervisor at two Chicago-area hospitals. After retirement, her love of writing brought freelance work with the *Chicago Tribune* and other publications.

Sherrie Kulwicki, R.N. ("Triumph in Trauma Room One"), lives in Paris, Texas, where she is a wife, mother, and registered nurse. The founder and president of Firmly Planted Ministries, Inc., she teaches and writes women's Bible studies, is a popular women's speaker, and has her own local televised Bible study series.

Lisa Lemming-Morton, R.N. ("The Last Dignity"), grew up in northwest Georgia and now lives in Ft. Myers, Florida, with her husband, John, and two children, ages six and eight. Currently an ER nurse, she has more than nine years experience in ICU, ER, and open heart ICU.

Cortney Martin ("Aunt Nurse") is a freelance writer living in Houston, Texas. Her published work ranges from fiction and creative nonfiction to award-winning journalism. She currently works as a public relations associate for a major nonprofit health-care organization serving the Texas Gulf Coast.

Robin O'Neal Matson ("Nurse Radar") is a single mother of three fascinating children, ages nine through fourteen. She coauthored *FlashPoint: Mastering the Art of Economic Abundance* and has developed programs on parenting and financial abundance. A writer, poet, and keeper of family history, her mission is to help adolescents envision healthy, meaningful futures.

Roberta McReynolds ("Room 108") balances her life with work, volunteering, writing, and hobbies. She donates time as a grief support group facilitator for children, and as a family visitor for hospice, she provides companionship for hospice patients and relief to their caregivers.

Mary Walsh Morello, R.N. ("Providence"), lives in Morton Grove, Illinois. She has been a nurse for twenty-five years, primarily in the emergency department. She has attended Northwestern University to further her writing career.

Marcella M. O'Malley ("Specialing Lieutenant Mulkerne") caught the writing bug while studying literature at the National University of Ireland. She currently lives in Wisconsin with her husband, Michael, and two great kids. Marcella has authored numerous short stories and is currently working on her second novel. The Mulkernes are her sister-in-law, Joanne's, parents.

Marie Golden Partain, R.N. ("Full Circle"), resides in Starr, South Carolina, with her husband of forty years. Currently employed as a certified psychiatric nurse with the South Carolina Department of Mental Health, she uses her writing therapeutically for her patients and herself. She also enjoys writing for her children and grandchildren.

Mary Ellen Porrata, R.N., A.P.R.N. ("Flight of the Gypsy King"), worked as an R.N. in the Boston area for over fifteen years, later obtaining a master's degree in nursing as an adult nurse practitioner. Married, with two grown sons, she currently studies and teaches mind-body medicine and yoga in Connecticut and enjoys writing about life experiences.

Terry Jean Ratner, R.N. ("Relinquishing a Soul"), works as a freelance writer and as a registered nurse at a level-one trauma hospital in Phoenix, Arizona. In June 2004, she received her Master of Fine Arts degree in creative nonfiction from Antioch University, Los Angeles. She has published numerous personal essays and writes book reviews for two national nursing publications.

Donna Surgenor Reames, R.N. ("A Measure of Worth"), mother of Zoe, Chloe, and Caroline, has been a registered nurse for twenty-two years. Currently a psychiatric nurse at an inpatient acute unit for children and adolescents at Medical University of South Carolina, Charleston, she is pursuing a master's degree and psychiatric nurse practitioner's license at MUSC. She has been writing freelance since 1986, and has been published in numerous publications, including *Brain, Child: The Magazine for Thinking Mothers*, *ADDitude magazine*, *CHILD magazine*, *The Front Porch*, and others.

Kimberly Ripley ("Hubba Hubba") lives and writes in New Hampshire with her husband and five children. She is the author of six books. Her "Freelancing Later in Life" workshop has inspired many new writers.

Shelia Bolt Rudesill, R.N. ("Do You Believe in Magic?" and "Macgillicuddy"), resides with her artist husband, Bud, in Chapel Hill, North Carolina, where she is a full-time NICU nurse. Her need to write stems from empathy for people who are burdened with unreasonable hardships. Shelia is the author of two novels: *Precious Children, Coveted Child* and *Auspicious Dreams*.

Shannon Shelton Rulé ("Something More for Margaret") resides in Starkville, Mississippi. A paralegal, writer, and children's storyteller, she favors inspirational, humor, and memoir writing. Her short stories and devotionals are published in several books and periodicals.

Carol Sharpe ("A Little Love Will Do It"), a semiretired long-term-care (LTC) nursing assistant, has worked as a freelance writer since receiving her creative writing diploma in 1996. Her writing has been published in anthologies, magazines, and newspapers. She and her husband live in British Columbia, Canada, where she competes in billiards.

Constance R. Shelsky, R.N., C.C.R.N. ("On the Other Side of the Bed"), and her husband live in Iowa. She is employed as a research nurse in the ICU of a local hospital but still works at the bedside from time to time.

Elizabeth Bussey Sowdal, R.N. ("Wherefore Art Thou, Julia?"), lives in Oklahoma City with her husband and four children. She is a staff nurse in the surgical-trauma intensive care unit at OU Medical Center and a freelance writer. With a busy household and an interesting job, she has plenty to write about.

Joyce Stark ("Divine Intervention") lives in northeast Scotland, where she works for the community mental health team. She writes for various publications in the United States and the United Kingdom, and is currently working on a series of stories for young children.

Mary E. Stassi, R.N.C. ("R$_x$ for the Best Worst Christmas"), is the health occupations coordinator at St. Charles Community College in St. Peters, Missouri. A seasoned nursing educator, textbook author, and well-known speaker, Mary lives with her husband, daughter, and five horses on a farm near St. Louis, Missouri.

Barbara Thatcher ("That Special Touch") is a freelance writer, retired bank internal auditor, and elder in her church. Her work has been published in *Angels on Earth* and *Route 66* magazines. Married for fifty-six years, she and her husband enjoy two daughters and twelve grandchildren, and live among the corn and soybean fields of central Illinois with their cat, Joe.

Elizabeth Turner, R.N. ("The Night Al Heel Broke Loose"), lives in Ontario, Canada.

Dorothy Wright, R.N. ("Cloudy with a Chance of Sunshine" and "Lady in Red"), currently resides in Manitoba, Canada, with her husband and two sons. Throughout her nursing career, Dorothy has treasured the little life lessons that patients share with her.

The *Cup of Comfort* Series!

All titles are $9.95 unless otherwise noted.

A Cup of Comfort
1-58062-524-X

A Cup of Comfort Cookbook ($12.95)
1-58062-788-9

A Cup of Comfort for Christmas
1-58062-921-0

A Cup of Comfort Devotional ($12.95)
1-59337-090-3

A Cup of Comfort Devotional for Women ($12.95)
1-59337-409-7

A Cup of Comfort for Friends
1-58062-622-X

A Cup of Comfort for Inspiration
1-58062-914-8

A Cup of Comfort for Mothers and Daughters
1-58062-844-3

A Cup of Comfort for Mothers and Sons
1-59337-257-4

A Cup of Comfort for Sisters
1-59337-097-0

A Cup of Comfort for Teachers
1-59337-008-3

A Cup of Comfort for Women
1-58062-748-X

A Cup of Comfort for Women in Love
1-59337-362-7

About the Editor

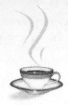

Colleen Sell is the editor of thirteen volumes in the *Cup of Comfort* anthology series. During her long career in words, she has been a book author, editor, and ghostwriter; magazine editor and features writer; journalist; tech writer; and copywriter.

She shares a big old house on a lavender farm in the Pacific Northwest with her husband, T.N. Trudeau, where she continues to weave stories both tall and true.